Dr.Ramiro Campos

COMPENDIUM OF OCCUPATIONAL AUDIOLOGY

Dr.Ramiro Campos

COMPENDIUM OF OCCUPATIONAL AUDIOLOGY

An analysis from practice

ScienciaScripts

Imprint

Any brand names and product names mentioned in this book are subject to trademark, brand or patent protection and are trademarks or registered trademarks of their respective holders. The use of brand names, product names, common names, trade names, product descriptions etc. even without a particular marking in this work is in no way to be construed to mean that such names may be regarded as unrestricted in respect of trademark and brand protection legislation and could thus be used by anyone.

Cover image: www.ingimage.com

This book is a translation from the original published under ISBN 978-3-639-73186-6.

Publisher:
Sciencia Scripts
is a trademark of
Dodo Books Indian Ocean Ltd. and OmniScriptum S.R.L publishing group

120 High Road, East Finchley, London, N2 9ED, United Kingdom
Str. Armeneasca 28/1, office 1, Chisinau MD-2012, Republic of Moldova, Europe
Printed at: see last page
ISBN: 978-620-6-07041-2

COMPENDIUM OF AUDIOLOGY
OCCUPATIONAL

AN ANALYSIS FROM PRACTICE
AUTHOR: RAMIRO CAMPOS
PROFESSOR RAMIRO CAMPOS

CONTENT

INTRODUCTION TO OCCUPATIONAL HEALTH

Occupational health refers to the discipline concerned with promoting and maintaining the physical, mental and social well-being of workers in their work environment. There are different models and approaches used in the field of occupational health, some of which include:

Occupational Accident Prevention Model: Focuses on identifying and eliminating occupational hazards that can cause injuries.

or illnesses in workers. This model is based on hazard identification, risk assessment and the implementation of control measures to prevent accidents and promote a safe working environment.

Health Promotion Model: Focuses on promoting healthy lifestyles and improving the general well-being of workers. This model is based on education and the promotion of healthy habits, such as a balanced diet, regular exercise, stress management and the prevention of work-related chronic diseases.

Ergonomic Evaluation Model: Focuses on adapting the work environment and workstations to the capabilities and needs of workers. Ergonomics seeks to optimize the relationship between people, equipment, tasks and the work environment, with the aim of improving efficiency, preventing musculoskeletal injuries and improving overall well-being.

Multidisciplinary Intervention Model: This model is based on collaboration between different occupational health professionals, such as physicians, nurses, psychologists, ergonomists and occupational safety experts. These professionals work together to identify and address occupational hazards, promote health and wellness, and provide interventions specific to individual needs and the work environment.

These are just some examples of models used in occupational health. It is important to note that models may vary according to the country, the organization and the specific circumstances of each work environment. Moreover, occupational health is constantly evolving, adapting to new risks and challenges in the world of work.

THE CODE OF HAMMURABI 1700 BC

The Code of Hammurabi is one of the oldest known sets of laws in human history. It was promulgated by King Hammurabi of Babylon around 1750 BC. The code consists of 282 laws covering a wide range of subjects, from trade and property to marriage and the family. These laws were intended to regulate the daily life and conduct of citizens in the ancient kingdom of Babylon.The Code of Hammurabi was inscribed on a stone stele, known as the Stele of Hammurabi, found in Susa, Iran, in the 12th century B.C. The text of the laws is written in cuneiform script, using the Akkadian language. The stele shows a representation of King Hammurabi receiving the laws from the god Shamash, the Babylonian god of justice.The Code of Hammurabi follows a principle of retributive justice, where the penalty or punishment for a crime is based on the principle of "an eye for an eye, a tooth for a tooth". However, it also establishes rules for the protection of the most vulnerable, such as widows, orphans and slaves. In addition, it addresses issues related to commerce, property, contracts, women's rights, marriage, divorce and professional responsibility.The Code of Hammurabi had a lasting influence on the history of law. Its legal and ethical principles laid the foundation for many later legal systems in different cultures. However, it also reflects the social structure and values of ancient Babylon, where there was a clear hierarchy and differential justice for different social classes.In summary, the Code of Hammurabi is an important historical document that represents one of the earliest legal codifications in human civilization. Although some of its laws may seem archaic or unjust from a modern perspective, it remains a valuable testimony to social organization and justice in ancient Babylon.

1778 AND THE EDICT OF CHARLES III

The Edict of Charles III of 1778, also known as the Edict of Free Trade, was an economic and political measure chosen by King Charles III of Spain. This edict sought to boost trade and the economy of the Spanish empire by relaxing trade restrictions and promoting freedom of commerce. The edict was based on a series of economic reforms implemented during the reign of Charles III, who aimed to modernize and strengthen the empire's economy. Among the main provisions of the edict were:Elimination of trade restrictions: Numerous decrees and regulations limiting trade, both internal and external, were repealed. The free circulation of goods within Spanish territory was allowed and tariffs and trade barriers were reduced.Stimulation of foreign trade: Trade with other countries was encouraged, especially those with which Spain had commercial treaties. The export of Spanish products was promoted and the import of goods necessary for the country's economy and industry was encouraged.Establishment of consulates: Consulates were created in different cities, both in Spain and in other countries, to facilitate trade and provide support to Spanish traders abroad.Promotion of agriculture and industry: The modernization and development of agriculture and industry in Spain was promoted. Incentives and support were granted to farmers and industrialists to improve production and product quality.Charles III's Edict of 1778 was an important measure that sought to boost the Spanish economy and strengthen the empire's trade. While it had a positive impact in some respects, it also had a negative impact in others.limitations and was unable to completely reverse the problems and political issues facing Spain at the time.In general, the edict reflected Charles III's concern to modernize the Spanish economy and adapt it to the changing demands of international trade. It was part of a set of reforms implemented during his reign that laid the groundwork for future economic and political changes in Spain.

XVI XVII CENTURY AND BERNARDINO RAMMAZINNI

Bernardino Ramazzini was a 17th century physician considered one of the pioneers in the field of occupational medicine and occupational disease prevention.Bernardino Ramazzini's legacy in occupational medicine is significant. His studies and writings influenced generations of physicians and laid the foundation for the development of occupational health policies and the protection of workers' rights. His preventive approach and his vision of occupational medicine as a specific discipline continue to be relevant today.In 1700, Ramazzini published his work "De Morbis Artificum Diatriba" (Treatise on the Diseases of Workers), which is considered the first systematic description of work-related diseases. In his work, Ramazzini identified and described a wide range of diseases affecting different groups of workers, including miners, metallurgists, farmers, potters, textile workers, and others.Ramazzini made detailed observations on the working conditions, occupational hazards and symptoms of diseases in each occupation. He recognized that many illnesses were caused by exposure to toxic substances, repetitive work, forced postures and other adverse working conditions.His work laid the foundation for the study of occupational diseases and the importance of prevention in the workplace. Ramazzini emphasized the need to identify and eliminate occupational hazards, as well as to provide protective and educational measures for workers.The history of occupational health, also known as occupational medicine or occupational health, dates back several centuries. The following is a summary of important milestones and developments in the history of occupational health around the world:Ancient Rome and Greece: Already in ancient times, some concerns about workers' health were evident. Hippocrates, considered the father of medicine, made observations about work-related diseases and recommended preventive measures.Industrial Revolution (18th century): With the advent of the Industrial Revolution, working conditions deteriorated significantly. Workers were exposed to long working hours, unhealthy environments, dangerous machinery and lack of protection. This led to an increase in occupational accidents and work-related diseases.Nineteenth century: In the mid-19th century, the first movements in favor of occupational health and safety emerged. In 1833, the "Factory Act" was passed in the United Kingdom, establishing regulations to improve working conditions in factories. In 1871, Germany was the first country to establish industrial accident insurance.Twentieth century: During the 20th century, significant advances in occupational health took place. In 1919, the International Labor Organization (ILO) was established, which promoted labor standards and workers' rights at the international level. In the 1950s, the first occupational health associations and societies were founded. Laws and regulations were introduced to protect workers from occupational hazards, occupational health services were established, and prevention and rehabilitation programs were developed.Today, occupational health continues to evolve to adapt to the changing challenges of the work environment. The prevention of occupational diseases and injuries is promoted, as well as the promotion of healthy work environments. Research is being conducted on new occupational hazards, such as those related to chemical exposure, occupational stress and ergonomics.At the global level, specialized occupational health organizations and agencies have been established, such as the ILO and the World Health Organization (WHO), which work to promote occupational health and safety worldwide and set international standards.The history of occupational health is a history of advances in the protection of workers' health and safety. Over the centuries, significant improvements in working conditions have been achieved and greater awareness of occupational hazards has been promoted. However, challenges remain, and work continues to ensure safe and healthy working environments for all workers.

THE HISTORY OF REBELLIOUS PATAGONIA

The "Patagonia Rebelde" is a historical episode that occurred in the Patagonia region of Argentina during the 1920s. It refers to a series of labor conflicts and violent repression that took place in the cattle industry and wool exploitation.The context of "Patagonia Rebelde" is set in a time of social and political change in Argentina. As the cattle industry developed in Patagonia, the workers of the región rural communities, mostly European and Creole immigrants, began to organize and demand better working conditions and fair wages.At that time, Patagonia was dominated by large estancias and powerful ranchers, who exploited rural workers in precarious conditions. Workers began to organize into unions and to carry out strikes and protests to demand better working conditions and union rights. The most emblematic conflict of the "Patagonia Rebelde" took place in the town of Puerto Deseado in 1921. There, the workers of the "Anita" ranch went on strike demanding wage increases and better working conditions. The response of the ranchers and the authorities was violent and repressive. The security forces brutally repressed the strike, mass arrests were made and summary trials were carried out.Repression continued in other parts of the region, such as the ranches of Santa Cruz and Tierra del Fuego. Cases of torture, summary executions and forced disappearances were recorded. The national government of the time, led by President Hipólito Yrigoyen, justified the repression by arguing that it was "anarchy" and an attempt at subversion.The "Patagonia Rebelde" conflict was harshly repressed and meant a defeat for rural workers and the trade union movement of the time. However, it left an important legacy in the struggle for labor rights and awareness of the need for union organization to improve working conditions.The history of "Rebel Patagonia" has been portrayed in several literary, cinematographic and theatrical works, such as Osvaldo Bayer's novel "La Patagonia Rebelde" and the film of the same name directed by Héctor Olivera. These works have contributed to keep alive the memory of this historical episode and to reflect on labor rights and workers' struggles in Argentina.

STUDIES

At international level, Gudelo Quintero & Hincapié Rubio (2021), in their research work called "Hearing loss caused by noise of occupational origin", aimed to analyze theoretically the hearing loss caused by noise of occupational origin. Documentary type research supported by a bibliographic design, the documentary sources were both physical and electronic, reviewed in the period from 2017 to 2020.

THE AUTHORS CONCLUDED THAT

Despite decades of research and its preventable nature, the incidence and prevalence of occupational noise-induced hearing loss is increasing, and all possible efforts for its prevention should be increased. Medicolegal aspects inherent to the compensation related to the damage caused by exposures in the work environment have been and continue to be one of the great challenges of this disease (p.30).The contribution of the study allows the presentation and depth of the subject, making it equally clear that it is important to have laws, but also to know how to implement them in conjunction with actions that help to create an adequate and safe work environment, as well as conditions that minimize risks to the hearing health of workers.In order to identify the risk factors present in the work environment that produce hearing loss in workers, Cerro Romero, Valladares Garrido et al. (2020) in their study entitled "Factors associated with noise-induced hearing loss in workers of a metal-mechanical company in Talara, Piura period 2015 -2018", conducted an investigation in which a population of five hundred and forty-three (543) workers was involved, data were taken from medical records collected by the company such as age, gender, medical history and frequency of noise in the studied environment.In concluding this study, the author highlights that there was no relationship between age and history of occupational disease and that there was a low prevalence of noise-induced hearing loss. In this case, he did as a recommendation, to perform annual audiometry tests, focusing mainly on the professional history associated with noise-induced hearing loss.The contribution of this study allows us to deepen the theoretical basis, in particular the relationship between the different individual conditions of workers, age, gender, risk factor, length of service and duration of exposure to noise in the presence of occupational noise-induced hearing loss.In a cross-sectional descriptive study with analytical character by Báez Rufino & Villalba Engel (2018), titled "Noise-induced hearing loss in workers exposed at work", where a survey was applied to one hundred and nine (109) employees of media companies in the city of Asunción in 2017, aimed to identify the occupational risks to which workers are exposed to noise.The author points out that workers exposed to noise have a significant risk of hearing loss, depending on exposure, daily workload and, given the irreversible nature of the people involved, it is necessary to improve the monitoring of preventive measures.This study is linked to the present research, generating contributions to the contextualization of the problem, as well as to the study variables related to noise-induced hearing loss and related factors, among others. At the national level, Bonilla Martínez (2020), in his work entitled "Exposure to noise associated with occupational diseases in workers of Confecciones Topy, S.A.", had the following resultsThe purpose of this study was to recognize noise pollution related to occupational diseases among workers of Confecciones Topy, S.A. The methodology was descriptive and applied, supported by a cross-sectional and documentary field project. The population involved was twenty (20) workers in the production area.In conclusion, the author states that, in order to prevent hearing disorders caused by exposure to noise in the work environment, a risk assessment is first required, a process that must be continuously monitored and, if necessary, controlled and modified. Based on this, it is estimated, the identification of the workplace, the existing risks and the list of affected workers, the appropriate preventive measures, among others.As a consequence of noise exposure, the most common occupational diseases are deafness, sleep disorders, tiredness and fatigue, tinnitus or ringing in the ears, noise-induced hearing loss, which causes a gradual and progressive hearing loss over time and is a totally irreversible disease. This study made contributions to the methodological aspect regarding the type and design of the study and the procedure to determine the areas and workplaces where workers are most exposed to noise.In a study conducted by Quintero Arosemena (2019), entitled "Noise level as an occupational risk factor at Hospital Santo Tomás and its impact on the health of workers in areas with excessive noise", the main objective was to describe the existing situation in the study facility, by evaluating the noise levels to which workers are exposed. The sample was made randomly, considering the workers in the otoscopy, scanning audiometry and soundproof booth audiometry rooms who subsequently underwent a reevaluation and were given a questionnaire on the same day.In a study conducted by Quintero Arosemena (2019), entitled "Noise level as an occupational risk factor in the Santo Tomás Hospital and its impact on the health of workers in areas with excessive noise", the objective was to describe the existing situation in the study facility, by evaluating the noise levels to which workers are exposed. The sample was randomly selected, considering the workers in the otoscopy, scanning audiometry and audiometry rooms in soundproof booths, who were subsequently reevaluated and a questionnaire was applied on the same day. The conclusions reached underline the importance of implementing an occupational health noise management program at the Santo Tomás Hospital, Panama City.Tovar Méndez (2018), in his work entitled "Relación existente entre el diagnóstico y t ipo de lesión auditiva en trabajadores expuestos al ruido en una empresa termoeléctrica", with the objective of determining the relationship between the occupational risk factor of industrial noise, the time of exposure and the degree of hearing damage in workers of a thermoelectric company. The nature of the study was descriptive and retrospective. The population studied comprised one hundred and seventy-eight workers. (178) employees.In conclusion, the author pointed out that the longer the duration of exposure to noise during work, the worse the audiological results obtained in the tests applied. In addition, he pointed out that people who are exposed to noise have an increased risk of hearing loss than those who are not. Therefore, it is necessary to implement a program of detection, measurement, evaluation and control of noise for the operators of the thermoelectric company, to determine the level of exposure of workers by the unsafe working condition to noise levels exceeding 85 decibels. The background information presented above has allowed us to present relevant and direct data and considerations related to the subject of the study, constituting a support and argument for some of the aspects of this research, either in terms of the approach to the problem, theoretical bases or methodology.

AUDIOLOGY

Audiology is a health care discipline that deals with the study, evaluation, diagnosis and treatment of hearing and balance disorders. Clinical audiology professionals, known as clinical audiologists, work with people of all ages, from newborns to older adults.The field of occupational audiology encompasses a wide range of areas including:Hearing evaluation: Clinical audiologists use a variety of tests and techniques to evaluate a person's hearing ability. These tests may include tonal audiometry,audiometry, impedance tests, otoacoustic emissions, among others. These evaluations help determine the degree and type of hearing loss present.Hearing aid fitting and selection: Clinical audiologists are trained to recommend and fit hearing devices, such as hearing aids, for those individuals with hearing loss. They perform verification and validation testing to ensure that hearing aids are properly fitted and provide adequate amplification.Aural rehabilitation: Clinical audiologists also work in aural rehabilitation programs, helping people with hearing loss adapt to and effectively use their hearing devices. They provide guidance and training on the use and care of hearing aids, communication strategies and management of difficult listening situations.Evaluation and management of balance disorders: Clinical audiologists can evaluate and treat balance-related disorders such as vertigo and dizziness. They use specific tests, such as videonystagmography (VNG) and posturography, to assess vestibular function and develop appropriate treatment plans.Education and prevention: Clinical audiologists play an important role in education and prevention of hearing loss. They provide information about the risks of exposure to excessive noise and promote hearing protection measures, such as the use of earplugs in noisy environments.

Occupational Audiology

Occupational audiology is a subspecialty of audiology that focuses on the evaluation of hearing related to the work environment and the prevention of occupational hearing loss. Occupational audiologists work in collaboration with occupational health professionals to identify, assess and mitigate hearing hazards in the workplace. The main objective of occupational audiology is to protect the hearing health of workers exposed to excessive noise or other auditory risk factors in their work environment. Some of the activities and areas of focus in occupational audiology include: Noise exposure assessment: Occupational audiologists make accurate noise level measurements in the workplace using specialized equipment. These measurements help determine whether workers are exposed to noise levels that could damage their hearing.

Hearing evaluation: Occupational audiologists perform hearing tests to evaluate the hearing function of workers exposed to occupational noise. These tests are used to detect hearing loss early and monitor any changes in hearing over time.Hearing conservation programs: Occupational audiologists develop and implement hearing conservation programs in the workplace. These programs include education on hearing hazards, proper use of hearing protection, hearing monitoring and promotion of safe practices to prevent occupational hearing loss.Recommendations and fitting of hearing protectors: Occupational audiologists advise workers on the proper selection, use and maintenance of hearing protectors, such as earplugs or earmuff-type hearing protectors. They also perform fit tests to ensure effective hearing protection.Research and development: Occupational audiologists are involved in research related to the prevention of occupational hearing loss, the effectiveness of hearing protectors and other areas related to hearing health in the workplace. Occupational audiology is essential to protect the hearing health of workers and ensure a safe working environment. Working closely with other occupational health professionals, occupational audiologists contribute to the early identification of occupational hearing loss and the implementation of appropriate preventive and protective measures.

Disease prevention

Health prevention refers to actions and strategies designed to avoid the appearance, development or spread of diseases and to promote people's general wellbeing. The main objective of health prevention is to prevent or reduce risk factors and promote healthy habits to keep people healthy and avoid the onset of disease.

There are different levels of health prevention:

Primary prevention: Focuses on preventing the onset of disease and promoting general health. Primary prevention measures include the promotion of healthy lifestyles, such as a balanced diet, regular physical activity, avoiding the consumption of alcohol, tobacco and other drugs. and alcohol, and vaccination. It also involves health education and awareness of risk factors and how to prevent them. Secondary prevention: Focuses on detecting and treating diseases in their early stages, when they have not yet caused serious symptoms. This involves screening and early diagnostic tests, such as mammograms, colon cancer screening, Pap smears, among others. The goal is to identify and treat diseases in their early stages to improve treatment outcomes and reduce morbidity and mortality.Tertiary prevention: Focuses on reducing the impact of a chronic disease or long-term disability. Tertiary prevention focuses on chronic disease management, rehabilitation, ongoing medical care, and emotional and social support to improve the quality of life of people who already have a chronic disease.

Health prevention strategies may include:

• Health awareness and education campaigns.
• Access a services from carehealth care preventive health care, such as vaccinations and screenings.
• Promotion of habits of lifestyles healthy lifestyles, such as a balanced diet and regular physical activity
• Public health policies, such as tobacco and alcohol restrictions.
• A safe and healthy work environment, including the management of occupational hazards.
• Control of diseases communicable diseases, such as measures and vector control measures.

Prevention in health is fundamental to reduce the burden of disease and promote a healthy lifestyle. By taking preventive measures, avoidable diseases can be prevented and people's quality of life can be improved. In addition, health prevention also has a positive impact on the health care system. by reducing the demand for medical care and the costs of health care. associated costs.

PREVENTION

Health prevention refers to actions and strategies designed to avoid the appearance, development or spread of diseases and to promote people's general wellbeing. The main objective of health prevention is to prevent or reduce risk factors and promote healthy habits to keep people healthy and avoid the onset of diseases.

There are different levels of health prevention:

Primary prevention: Focuses on preventing the onset of disease and promoting general health. Primary prevention measures include the promotion of healthy lifestyles, such as a balanced diet, regular physical activity, avoidance of tobacco and alcohol consumption, and vaccination. It also involves health education and awareness of risk factors and how to prevent them.
Secondary prevention : Focuses on detecting and treating diseases in their early stages, when they have not yet caused serious symptoms. This involves screening and early diagnostic tests, such as mammograms, colon cancer screening, Pap smears, among others. The goal is to identify and treat diseases in their early stages to improve treatment outcomes and reduce morbidity and mortality.

Tertiary prevention: Focuses on reducing the impact of a chronic disease or long-term disability. Tertiary prevention focuses on chronic disease management, rehabilitation, ongoing medical care, and emotional and social support to improve the quality of life of people who already have a chronic disease.

Prevention of hearing loss

Preventing hearing loss is critical to preserving hearing health throughout life. Here are some key measures and practices to prevent hearing loss: Hearing protection in noisy environments: Avoid prolonged exposure to loud noise and use hearing protection, such as earplugs or earmuffs, in noisy environments such as concerts, noisy workplaces, sporting events or during the use of noisy power tools.Volume control on sound reproduction devices: Limit the volume and time of exposure to sound reproduction devices such as music players, cell phones, televisions and headphones. Avoid listening to music at high volumes for prolonged periods of time and consider using noise-canceling headphones to reduce the need to increase the volume.Education and awareness: Learn about the risks of noise exposure and the importance of protecting your hearing. Know the safe limits of noise exposure and share this information with others, especially younger people, to encourage safe sound practices. Get regular hearing tests: Get regular hearing tests, especially if you work in noisy environments or if you have additional risk factors, such as a family history of hearing loss or diseases that can affect hearing. Hearing tests can detect any signs of hearing loss early and allow for appropriate preventive measures or treatment.Avoid using cotton swabs in the ears: Avoid inserting objects such as cotton swabs or other devices into the ear canal, as they can damage the ear and push wax into the eardrum, which can cause blockage or injury. Promoting a safe working environment: Employers should implement noise control measures in the workplace and provide adequate hearing protection equipment. In addition, training and awareness programs on the importance of hearing protection and safe noise practices should be established.Remember that prevention is key, as noise-induced hearing loss is largely irreversible. By taking proactive steps to protect your hearing and adopting healthy sound-related lifestyle habits, you can minimize the risk of hearing loss and maintain healthy hearing over time.

Communication at risk

Communication in risk or emergency situations is crucial to ensure the safety and well-being of those affected. In these situations, effective communication can help inform, educate and guide people about hazards, safety measures and actions to take.

Here are some key points related to communication in the following areas risk situations:Clear and accurate information: Communication should provide clear, accurate and easily understandable information on the nature of the risk, safety measures and recommended actions. It is important to use simple language and avoid technical terms or jargon that may cause confusion.Multiple communication channels: It is essential to use different communication channels to reach as many people as possible. This may include the use of public address systems, radios, text messages, social networks, websites, media, among others. Messages should be adapted to the channel used and take into account the limitations of each one.Constant updating: Information should be updated regularly as the situation evolves and new information becomes available. Affected persons need to be aware of changes in risks, security measures and instructions. Transparency and open communication help to build trust and credibility in the authorities or sources of information.

Active listening and feedback: Communication should be two-way, allowing people to ask questions, express concerns, and provide feedback. Authorities and those responsible for communication should be prepared to actively listen, respond to questions, and address the information needs of affected people.Adaptation to diversity: Communication should be inclusive and consider the needs of different groups of people, such as people with disabilities, people from different cultures and people who speak different languages. It is important to use different formats, such as images, graphics, captions or sign language interpretation, as needed.

Coordination and collaboration: Effective communication in risk situations requires close coordination and collaboration between different actors, such as government agencies, emergency response organizations, the media, and the community at large. All must work together to ensure that messages are consistent and disseminated appropriately.

Communication in situations of risk is essential to inform and protect the people affected. Clear, up-to-date, two-way communication adapted to the needs of the diversity of people is essential to ensure safety and well-being in these circumstances.

TYPOLOGY OF OCCUPATIONAL HAZARDS

It is important that employers identify and assess specific occupational hazards in their workplaces and take measures to control and prevent them. This involves implementing safety measures, providing adequate training, offering personal protective equipment, promoting safe practices, and fostering a culture of safety in the workplace.Within the work environment there are several types of risks, among which are the followingPhysical risks: These risks include exposure to intense noise, vibrations, ionizing radiation (such as X-rays and radiotherapy), non-ionizing radiation (such as ultraviolet light), extreme temperatures (cold or heat), inadequate lighting, electricity, fire and explosions.Chemical hazards: These refer to exposure to hazardous chemicals, such as toxic chemicals, gases, vapors, fumes, dusts and solvents. These chemicals can enter the body through inhalation, ingestion or skin contact and can cause'illness, poisoning or allergic reactions.Biological hazards: These hazards are associated with exposure to living organisms, such as bacteria, viruses, fungi, parasites and biological toxins. They can occur in healthcare settings, laboratories, agriculture, waste treatment and other industries where there is contact with biological materials.Ergonomic risks: These are related to the way jobs, equipment and working conditions are organized. They include repetitive movements, awkward postures, manual lifting and carrying of loads, intense physical effort, inadequate design of equipment and furniture, and psychosocial factors such as work stress.Psychosocial risks: These risks affect the mental and emotional health of workers. They may include high workloads, lack of control over tasks, lack of social support, lack of clarity in roles and responsibilities, workplace harassment, workplace violence, and emotional demands.Safety risks: These risks relate to situations or conditions that may cause accidents or physicalinjuries. They include unsafe working conditions, lack of adequate personal protective equipment (PPE), lack of safety training, risk of falls, entrapment, cuts, blows, and injuries related to the use of machinery and tools.

Occupational health management

Health services management refers to the planning, organization, coordination, and supervision of medical and health care services. The main objective of health services management is to ensure the effective and efficient provision of quality health services to meet patient needs and improve health outcomes. Here are some key areas of health services management:Strategic planning: Health services management involves developing a strategic vision and defining goals and objectives for the health care organization. This includes identifying the health needs of the population, assessing available resources, and planning the services needed to address those needs.Occupational health management refers to the management and promotion of health and safety in the work environment. Its main objective is to ensure that workers are protected from occupational hazards and that their well-being at work is promoted. Here are some key areas of occupational health management:Financial management: Health services management involves managing the financial resources of the health care organization. This involves developing and monitoring budgets, managing costs, and seeking sources of financing to ensure the economic sustainability of health services.Quality management: Health services management focuses on ensuring the quality of health care services. This includes setting quality standards, implementing quality control systems, monitoring patient safety, measuring outcomes, and implementing continuous improvement in the quality of services.Information and technology management: Health services management involves the efficient management of information and technology in the healthcare environment. This includes the implementation and management of health information systems, the use of medical and digital technology, and ensuring the security and confidentiality of patient data.Patient relationship management: Health services management is concerned with establishing and maintaining a good relationship with patients. This includes effective communication with patients, patient-centered care, complaint and grievance management, and improving the patient experience in the healthcare organization.Healthcare management is essential to ensuring the effective delivery of quality healthcare services. By efficiently managing resources, promoting quality and safety, and focusing on patient needs, healthcare organizations can achieve better health outcomes and patient satisfaction.Human resource management: Health services management involves the management of the health care organization's personnel. This includes the recruitment and training of healthcare professionals, staffing, performance evaluation, talent management, and the promotion of a healthy and collaborative work environment.Risk assessment: Occupational health management involves identifying and assessing the risks present in the work environment. This includes conducting risk assessments and safety analyses to determine the conditions and activities that could endanger the health and safety of workers.Development of policies and procedures: Occupational health management involves establishing clear policies and procedures related to occupational health and safety. These policies should address aspects such as accident prevention, protection against chemical, physical and biological hazards, promotion of health and well-being, and compliance with applicable regulations and standards. Implementation of control measures: Occupational health management is responsible for implementing control measures to minimize or eliminate occupational hazards. This may include the implementation of technical controls, such as modifications in the design of equipment and machinery, as well as the use of personal protective equipment (PPE) and appropriate training in its use.Training and awareness: Occupational health management involves providing training and awareness to employees on occupational hazards and prevention measures. This includes informing them about the risks associated with their work, how they can be to properly use personal protective equipment and safe work practices, as well as educate on the importance of maintaining good health and wellness in the work environment.Monitoring and compliance: Occupational health management involves regularly monitoring and evaluating the effectiveness of implemented health and safety measures. This may include conducting regular workplace inspections, monitoring exposure to hazardous substances, monitoring employee health, and ensuring compliance with relevant regulations and standards.Promoting health and well-being: In addition to addressing occupational hazards, occupational health management also promotes the health and well-being of workers. This may include implementing health promotion programs, promoting healthy lifestyles, managing work-related stress, and facilitating work-life balance. Occupational health management is fundamental to protecting the health and safety of workers, improving productivity and promoting a healthy work environment. By taking a proactive approach to identifying and controlling occupational hazards, organizations can ensure a safe and healthy work environment for their employees.

PAHO and occupational health

PAHO plays a key role in the promotion and protection of occupational health in the Americas region. It works closely with member countries, other international organizations, and key stakeholders to improve working conditions, prevent occupational hazards, and promote safe and healthy work environments.The Pan American Health Organization (PAHO) is a regional entity of the World Health Organization (WHO) responsible for promoting and protecting health in the Americas. In the area of occupational health, PAHO plays an important role in providing guidance, technical support and promotion of good occupational health practices in the region. Some of PAHO's activities and approaches in occupational health include Policy and regulatory development: PAHO works in collaboration with member countries to develop occupational health policies and regulations. This includes promoting laws and regulations that protect the health and safety of workers, and promoting rights-based approaches to labor.Strengthening surveillance systems: PAHO supports the implementation of epidemiological surveillance systems for work-related diseases and occupational injuries. This makes it possible to collect data and information on the incidence of occupational diseases and injuries, identify trends, and develop appropriate prevention strategies. Promotion of good practices: PAHO promotes the adoption of good practices in occupational health in the region. This includes the dissemination of information on prevention measures, the promotion of participatory approaches involving employers and workers, and the promotion of research and knowledge exchange in the field of occupational health.Training and capacity building: PAHO provides training and technical support to member countries in occupational health capacity building. This includes the training of health professionals and occupational health specialists, the promotion of occupational health education, and the training of health professionals in occupational health. education and awareness of occupational hazards, and strengthening the capacities of health systems to address the needs in this field.Technical cooperation and collaboration: PAHO promotes technical cooperation and collaboration among member countries in the field of occupational health. This includes the exchange of experiences and best practices, collaboration on joint projects and programs, and the mobilization of resources to support the implementation of occupational health measures.

Epistemology of health

Health epistemology is a discipline that analyzes the nature, production and application of knowledge in the field of health. It examines the theoretical and philosophical foundations underlying the generation and use of knowledge in health, and contributes to a deeper understanding of the health sciences.Health epistemology addresses questions related to the nature of knowledge in health, the different approaches to generating scientific evidence, the ways in which that knowledge is interpreted and applied, and the challenges and limitations associated with the production of knowledge in this field. Some important aspects of health epistemology include:Paradigms and research approaches: Health epistemology examines the different research paradigms and approaches used to generate knowledge in the health field. This may include quantitative, qualitative, and mixed approaches, as well as approaches based on evidence-based medicine, epidemiology, social sciences, and other related fields.Sources of knowledge: Health epistemology explores the different sources of knowledge used in health, such as scientific evidence, epidemiological data, clinical experience, traditional knowledge and patient perspectives.It examines how this diversity of knowledge sources is evaluated and integrated into health care decision making and practice. Validity and reliability of knowledge: Health epistemology investigates the criteria for assessing the validity and reliability of knowledge in the field of health. It examines how to establish the robustness of research, the replicability of studies, the quality of evidence, the consistency of results and other aspects related to the reliability of knowledge in health. Application of knowledge: Health epistemology considers how knowledge is applied and used in health decision-making and practice. It examines the processes of translating evidence into policy and practice, the challenges associated with implementing evidence-based interventions, and the relationship between scientific knowledge and the perspectives and values of patients and communities.Philosophical perspectives: The epistemology of health is based on diverse ph ilosophical perspectives that influence how health knowledge is conceived and constructed. This may include pragmatist, constructivist, realist, and critical approaches, among others, which influence conceptions of knowledge and debates about its production and use in health.

Public policies and health

Public policies on occupational health are the set of actions and decisions taken by governments and other governmental entities to promote and protect the health and safety of workers in the work environment. These policies aim to prevent work-related injuries, illnesses and deaths, and to promote safe and healthy working conditions. Some key areas of public policy in occupational health include:Labor legislation and regulations: Public policies on occupational health are based on the enactment of labor laws and regulations that establish the rights and responsibilities of employers and workers in relation to occupational health and safety. These regulations establish minimum standards for the protection of workers and may address issues such as risk prevention, the use of personal protective equipment, exposure to hazardous substances, and the organization of working time.Inspections and enforcement: Public policies on occupational health include the implementation of labor inspection programs to verify compliance with occupational health and safety rules and regulations. These inspections can be conducted on a regular basis and help ensure that employers comply with established standards and take the necessary measures to protect the health of their workers.Promotion of prevention: Public policies on occupational health promote the adoption of preventive measures in the work environment. This may include awareness and education campaigns on occupational hazards, promotion of safe work practices, training of employers and workers on occupational safety issues, and encouragement of workers' active participation in risk identification and prevention.Epidemiological surveillance: Public policies on occupational health involve the collection and analysis of epidemiological data on work-related diseases and injuries. This makes it possible to identify trends, evaluate the impact of working conditions on workers' health and guide prevention and control actions. Research and evidence development: Public policies on occupational health are based on scientific research and evidence development. This involves supporting research in the field of occupational health, collecting data on occupational hazards and their impact on health, and generating evidence to support the adoption of effective policies and prevention measures. Collaboration and coordination: Public policies on occupational health involve collaboration and coordination among different actors, including governments, employers, workers, unions, civil society organizations and academic institutions. These collaborations allow for a comprehensive approach to occupational health and safety protection.Public policies on occupational health are fundamental to guarantee the protection of workers and promote safe and healthy work environments. These policies are based on the recognition of labor rights.

Codes sanitary

The sanitary code is a set of legal norms and provisions that regulate public health and establish guidelines for the protection of the health of the population. The specific content and structure of the sanitary code may vary depending on the country or jurisdiction. The following are some common elements found in many sanitary codes:Regulation of sanitary practices: The sanitary code establishes requirements and regulations for various sanitary practices, such as hygiene, disease prevention, health promotion, epidemiological surveillance, control of communicable diseases, and management of health emergencies. Licenses and permits: The health code may require that certainfacilities and health care professionals obtain licenses and permits to operate. This may include hospitals, clinics, pharmacies, laboratories, food services, health care facilities and health care professionals, such as doctors, nurses and pharmacists.Regulation of medical devices: The health code may include regulations for the production, distribution and marketing of medical devices, such as drugs, medical devices, food and hazardous chemicals. This may cover aspects such as safety, efficacy, labeling, storage and transportation of these products.Public health protection: The sanitary code establishes measures for public health protection and disease prevention. This may include disease surveillance, mandatory reporting of communicable diseases, promotion of vaccination, food and water safety, and management of outbreaks and epidemics.Sanctions and enforcement: The sanitary code establishes sanctions and enforcement measures for those who violate sanitary provisions. This may include fines, suspensions, revocation of licenses, and other disciplinary measures to ensure compliance with regulations and protect public health. It is important to note that health codes can vary significantly between countries and jurisdictions. Each country has its own sanitary code, adapted to its specific public health context, needs and regulations.

Role of state

The state has the responsibility to establish and promote occupational health policies that protect the health and safety of workers. This involves the elaboration of laws and regulations, the supervision of compliance.The role of the state in occupational health policies is fundamental to ensure the protection of workers and promote safe and healthy work environments. Some of the responsibilities and functions that correspond to the state in this area includeLegislation and regulation: The state has the responsibility to establish laws and regulations that protect the health and safety of workers. These regulations establish the minimum standards that employers must comply with in terms of risk prevention, occupational hygiene, occupational safety, protection against hazardous substances, among other aspects. Legislation may also include provisions on the education and training of workers, the use of personal protective equipment and the organization of working time.Implementation and enforcement of regulations: The state must ensure that occupational health laws and regulations are effectively enforced. This involves carrying out labor inspections, monitoring compliance with established standards, and applying sanctions for noncompliance. It may also include the promotion of occupational safety and health management systems, the promotion of good practices, and education and awareness of occupational hazards. Epidemiological surveillance and occupational health statistics: The state has the responsibility to collect data and conduct epidemiological surveillance of work-related diseases and injuries. This involves collecting information on the incidence and prevalence of occupational diseases, occupational injuries, and other work-related health problems. These data are essential for identifying trends, assessing the impact of working conditions on workers' health, and guiding prevention policies and measures.Prevention and occupational health promotion: The state has a key role in promoting risk prevention and occupational health promotion. This may include the dissemination of information on best practices in occupational health and safety, the promotion of training and capacity-building programs for employers and workers, and raising awareness of occupational hazards and prevention measures. It may also include the promotion of policies and practices that encourage healthy work environments and the active participation of workers in risk identification and prevention.Cooperation and coordination: The state should foster cooperation and coordination among different actors, including employers, workers, unions, civil society organizations, and other entities related to occupational health. This implies establishing mechanisms for social dialogue, facilitating collaboration in the implementation of policies and programs, and promoting the participation of all stakeholders in decision making related to occupational health.

INDUSTRIAL HYGIENE AND OCCUPATIONAL HEALTH

Industrial hygiene and occupational health are two related disciplines that focus on protecting the health and safety of workers in the work environment, but they focus on slightly different aspects. Here I explain the difference between the two:

Industrial Hygiene:

Industrial hygiene focuses primarily on the identification, evaluation and control of physical, chemical and biological agents. present in the workplace that can cause illness or injury to workers.It is intended to prevent exposure to toxic or hazardous substances. and minimize the health risks associated with these agents.Industrial hygiene deals with the sampling and analysis of contaminants present in the work environment, the evaluation of workers' exposure to those contaminants, and the design and implementation of appropriate control measures to reduce or eliminate risks.Typical industrial hygiene activities include air quality assessment, noise measurement, lighting assessment, chemical and biological substance analysis, and implementation of engineering or administrative control strategies to minimize exposure.

Occupational Health:

Occupational health, also known as occupational medicine or occupational medicine, focuses on the well-being and general health of workers in relation to their work.Its objective is to prevent and treat work-related illnesses, injuries and disorders, as well as to promote a safe and healthy work environment.Occupational health encompasses a wide range of aspects, including injury prevention, health promotion, diagnosis and treatment of occupational diseases, monitoring of workers' health, and management of occupational disability.Typical occupational health activities include occupational medical examinations, occupational safety and health counseling, fitness-for-duty assessment, rehabilitation and return to work after injury or illness, and promotion of workers' health and well-being. In summary, industrial hygiene focuses on the identification and control of physical, chemical and biological agents present in the workplace, while occupational health encompasses a broader perspective that includes the diagnosis, prevention and treatment of work-related illnesses and injuries, as well as the promotion of a healthy work environment. Both disciplines are complementary and are combined to ensure the integral protection of workers in the work environment. Occupational health and industrial safety are two closely related disciplines that focus on protecting the health, safety and welfare of workers in the work environment. Although they share common objectives, there are some differences between them:

Occupational Health:

Occupational health is concerned with the promotion and maintenance of the physical, mental and social health of workers in relation to their work.Its main objective is to prevent and control occupational hazards, as well as to promote the health and general well-being of workers in their work environment.Occupational health includes activities such as occupational risk assessment, hazard identification and control, and the promotion of healthy practices and lifestyles in the workplace.It focuses on aspects such as ergonomics, occupational hygiene, occupational medicine, occupational mental health, health promotion and occupational disability management.

Industrial Safety:

Industrial safety focuses on preventing accidents and injuries in the workplace.Its main objective is to identify and control occupational hazards and risks to ensure a safe working environment and reduce the potential for injury, accident or property damage.Industrial safety includes activities such ,as hazard identification, risk assessment, design of safety management systems, safety training, use of personal protective equipment (PPE), implementation of control measures and emergency response.It focuses on aspects such as facility safety, safe handling of hazardous substances, fire and explosion prevention, and safety in the use of machinery and equipment.occupational health focuses on promoting the health and well-being of workers in relation to their work, while industrial safety focuses on preventing occupational accidents and injuries through the identification and control of hazards and risks. Both disciplines are complementary and work together to ensure a safe, healthy and productive work environment.

Public health vs. occupational health

Public health and occupational health are two related but distinct disciplines that deal with different aspects of people's health and well-being. Here are the differences between them:

Public Health:

Public health focuses on the health and well-being of populations in general, not only in the work environment.Its main objective is to prevent disease, promote health and improve the quality of life of communities. Public health addresses health problems at the population level, such as infectious diseases, chronic diseases, maternal and child health, environmental health, promotion of healthy lifestyles, emergency planning and response, among others.Public health interventions include health policies, health education, immunization programs, communicable disease control, access to health services, and community health assessment.

Occupational Health:

Occupational health focuses specifically on the health and safety of workers.well-being of workers in their work environment.Its main objective is to prevent work-related illnesses, injuries and disorders and to promote a safe and healthy work environment.Occupational health addresses specific aspects of work, such as exposure to toxic substances, noise, vibrations, ergonomic and psychosocial factors at work.Occupational health interventions include occupational risk assessment, implementation of engineering and administrative controls, promotion of safe work practices, occupational safety education and training, and worker health surveillance.Public health focuses on the health of general populations, addressing a wide range of health problems at the community level, while occupational health focuses on the health and safety of workers in their work environment, addressing specific work-related risks and challenges. Both disciplines are important in protecting the health and well-being of individuals, but with different approaches and scopes.

Noise and health

Noise can have a significant impact on people's health. Prolonged exposure to high noise levels can cause a range of health problems, both physical and psychological. Here are some key aspects about noise and its impact on healthHearing loss: Continuous exposure to high noise levels can damage the auditory system and cause hearing loss. Intense noise can damage the sensory cells of the inner ear, which can result in permanent and irreversible hearing loss. It is important to protect the ears from excessive noise exposure by wearing appropriate hearing protection. Sleep disorders: Constant loud noise can interfere with sleep and cause sleep disorders such as insomnia, difficulty falling asleep and frequent awakenings during the night. This can have a negative impact on quality of life, cognitive performance and overall health.Stress and mental health: Chronic exposure to noise can cause chronic stress, which in turn can have adverse effects on mental health. Constant, disruptive noise can cause irritability, anxiety, depression, difficulty concentrating, and other problems related to mood and emotional well-being.Cardiovascular problems: Long-term noise exposure has been associated with an increased risk of developing cardiovascular diseases, such as high blood pressure, heart disease, stroke and heart rhythm disorders. Chronic stress caused by noise is believed to play an important role in this association.

Other physical effects: In addition to hearing and mental health problems, noise exposure has also been linked to other physical effects, such as headaches, digestive discomfort, concentration problems, decreased cognitive performance and increased irritability.To prevent the negative health effects of noise, it is important to take control and protective measures. These may include reducing noise at the source, using appropriate hearing protection, designing sound-insulated work and living spaces, and implementing policies and regulations to control noise exposure in occupational and community settings.It is important to keep in mind that safe levels of noise exposure may vary according to the regulations and standards established in each country. It is advisable to follow the guidelines and recommendations of occupational and environmental health experts to protect your hearing and general health from the harmful effects of noise.

The sound

Sound is a form of energy that is produced when there is a vibration in a medium, such as air, water or solids. This vibration creates sound waves that propagate through the medium and can be perceived by the human ear or other sound detection devices.

Sound is characterized by several properties:

Frequency: It is the number of vibrations complete (cycles) that occur in one second and is measured in Hertz (Hz). The frequency determines the pitch of the sound, where high frequencies correspond to high-pitched sounds and low frequencies correspond to low-pitched sounds.Amplitude: This is the measure of the intensity or energy of the sound and is related to the perceived loudness. Amplitude is expressed in decibels (dB), where a higher amplitude corresponds to a louder sound.Timbre: The tonal quality of sound that allows different musical instruments or voices to be distinguished. Timbre is determined by the unique characteristics of the sound wave, such as shape and harmonic content.Sound can be produced by a variety of sources, including human voices, musical instruments, vehicles, machinery, animals and natural events such as thunder. These sources generate vibrations that propagate as sound waves through the medium, and when these waves reach the human ear, they are picked up by the auditory system and interpreted as sound.In addition to being perceived by the human ear, sound can also be measured and analyzed using specialized devices such as microphones and sound analyzers. These instruments can provide accurate measurements of the intensity, frequency and other characteristics of sound.Sound plays a crucial role in our lives, allowing us to communicate, perceive our surroundings, enjoy music and alert us to potential dangers. However, it is important to keep in mind that exposure to loud or prolonged sound can have negative effects on hearing and overall health, so it is necessary to take steps to protect our hearing and maintain a healthy sound environment.Noise and sound are related terms, but they have important differences in their meaning and connotation. Here I explain the difference between the two:Sound: Sound refers to vibrations that propagate through a medium (such as air, water, or solids) and can be perceived by the human ear or other sound detection devices. Sound can be pleasant, harmonic and musical, such as music, the human voice or natural sounds. Sound is characterized by properties such as frequency, amplitude and timbre, which determine its pitch, loudness and quality.Noise: Noise is unwanted, inharmonious or undesirable sound that interferes with communication, rest, concentration or other human activities. Noise is considered annoying, irritating or harmful to health when it exceeds certain levels or when its frequency or characteristics are not appropriate for the situation. Noise can be produced by sources such as industrial machinery, traffic, construction, loud voices, noisy appliances, among others.sound refers to audible and perceptible vibrations in a pleasant and harmonious manner, noise is characterized as an undesirable, annoying or harmful form of sound that adversely affects the quality of life and may have adverse health effects. The perception of sound and noise is subjective and may vary according to individual preferences and tolerances.It is important to keep in mind that prolonged exposure to high noise levels can cause hearing damage and other health problems, such as stress, sleep problems, concentration difficulties and disorders of the cardiovascular system. Therefore, it is essential to take hearing protection measures and reduce exposure to excessive noise to maintain good hearing and overall health.

The hearing study in human resources

The study of hearing in workers is an important part of occupational health. The main objective is to evaluate the hearing status of workers exposed to noise levels or other agents that may affect their hearing, and to take preventive measures to avoid hearing loss.occupational hearing loss. Some key aspects of the study of hearing in workers are presented here: Initial assessment: An initial hearing assessment is performed for workers exposed to noise levels or other agents that may damage hearing. This may include audiometric testing to measure the hearing ability of workers and establish a baseline.Periodic monitoring: Periodic monitoring of the hearing of exposed workers is carried out. This involves regular repetition of audiometric tests to evaluate any changes in hearing and to detect early signs of hearing loss. The frequency of monitoring depends on the standards and regulations established for the type of occupational exposure.

Risk identification: The study of hearing in workers also involves identifying and assessing specific hearing hazards present in the work environment. This may include measuring noise levels, identifying other agents harmful to hearing (such as ototoxic chemicals) and assessing work processes that may contribute to hearing exposure.Implementation of preventive measures: Based on the results of audiometric testing and risk assessment, preventive measures should be implemented to protect workers' hearing. This may include the implementation of engineering controls to reduce noise levels, the use of hearing protectors, hearing awareness training, and the promotion of a hearing safety culture in the workplace.Education and awareness: The study of hearing in workers also includes education and awareness of hearing hazards, preventive measures, and the importance of protecting hearing in the work environment. This involves providing information and training to workers on the effects of noise on hearing, how to properly use hearing protection, and safe work practices related to hearing. The study of hearing in workers is fundamental to identify and prevent occupational hearing loss. It involves initial assessment and periodic monitoring of hearing, identification of hazards, implementation of preventive measures, and education of workers. This helps to maintain a safe work environment and protect workers' hearing health.Hearing loss and deafness are terms used to describe hearing loss to varying degrees. Here is a description of both terms:

Hearing loss: Hearing loss refers to a decrease in hearing ability to any degree, whether mild, moderate, severe or profound. People with hearing loss may have difficulty hearing soft sounds or conversations in noisy environments. Hearing loss can be congenital (present from birth) or acquired due to various factors, such as exposure to noise, infections, diseases, trauma, among others. In some cases, hearing loss can be corrected or treated with the use of hearing aids, cochlear implants or other assistive listening devices.

Deafness: Deafness is a more significant hearing loss, generally classified as a severe or profound hearing loss. People with deafness have significant difficulty perceiving sounds and may have very limited or no hearing. Deafness can be congenital or acquired in origin, and can be caused by factors similar to those of hearing loss. People with deafness may benefit from cochlear implants or other treatment options, but it is important to note that profound deafness can have a significant impact on communication and may require other forms of communication, such as sign language. It is important to mention that hearing loss can have different degrees and causes, and each case is unique. It is recommended that individuals experiencing any type of hearing loss seek evaluation and treatment from hearing health care professionals. hearing health, as well as to determine the degree of hearing loss and explore appropriate treatment options .

Central auditory processing (CAP) refers to the way the brain receives, interprets and uses auditory information from the ears. It is a set of skills that allows the brain to analyze, organize and understand the sounds we perceive in our environment.

Central auditory processing involves different processes that occur in the central nervous system, from the brainstem to the higher auditory areas of the brain. These processes include:

Sound localization and lateralization: The brain is able to determine the direction from which a sound comes and to discriminate between sounds coming from different sources.

• Auditory discrimination: The brain can distinguish between different frequencies and characteristics of sounds, such as pitch, timbre and intensity.

• Auditory attention: The brain can focus on a specific sound while filtering out or ignoring other irrelevant or distracting sounds.

• Auditory memory: The brain can retain and remember the short- and long-term auditory information.

• Auditory and visual integration: The brain can combine auditory information with visual information for a more complete understanding of the environment.

Impaired central auditory processing can affect a person's ability to understand speech, follow directions, participate in conversations in noisy environments and adequately process environmental sounds. This can impact learning, language development and communication.

The evaluation of central auditory processing is performed by means of specific tests that assess different abilities mentioned above. The results of these tests can help identify deficiencies in central auditory processing and guide appropriate interventions and therapies.It is important to note that central auditory processing is a complex and multidimensional aspect of hearing, and difficulties in auditory processing can occur in varying degrees and in relation to a variety of conditions, such as developmental disorders, brain injury, language disorders, and autism spectrum disorders. Evaluation and treatment of central auditory processing is usually performed by professionals specializing in audiology or speech therapists and may include auditory therapy, training exercises and compensatory strategies to improve auditory processing skills.

Periodic audiometries

Audiometries are tests used to evaluate the hearing of workers exposed to noise levels in their work environments. These tests are an important part of occupational health hearing surveillance programs and aim to detect possible noise-induced hearing loss and take appropriate preventive measures. Here are some key aspects related to audiometry in workers: Purpose of audiometries: The main purpose of audiometries in workers is to evaluate hearing function and detect possible hearing loss caused by occupational noise exposure. These tests allow early identification of hearing changes and preventive measures to be taken before permanent hearing damage occurs.Frequency of audiometry: The frequency with which audiometries should be performed may vary according to the legislation and regulations of each country. Generally, it is recommended to perform a baseline audiometry before the worker begins to be exposed to significant noise levels. Thereafter, periodic follow-up audiometries are performed to detect any changes in hearing.Hearing evaluation: During an audiometry, audiometers are used to emit different tones and volumes into the worker's ears. The worker must indicate when he hears the sound and at what volume level. These results are compared with normal hearing levels to determine if there is any hearing loss and its degree of severity.
Interpretation of results: The results of an audiometry are presented on an audiogram, which shows the worker's hearing ability at different frequencies. A health care professional trained in audiology will interpret the results and determine if there is a significant hearing loss and if additional measures are needed to protect the worker's hearing health.
Subsequent actions: If hearing loss is detected, appropriate measures should be taken to protect the worker's hearing health and prevent further deterioration. This may include changes in the work environment to reduce noise exposure, providing hearing protection equipment, providing training on preventive measures, and promoting awareness of the importance of hearing health.It is important to note that audiometries should be performed by professionals trained in audiology and in compliance with the regulations and standards established by occupational health authorities. These tests are an important tool in monitoring the hearing health of workers exposed to noise levels in their work environments and contribute to the prevention and control of occupational hearing loss. The calibration of audiometers is of utmost importance in hearing evaluation, as it ensures the accuracy and reliability of the results obtained during audiometric testing. Some key reasons for the importance of audiometer calibration are highlighted below: Accuracy of measurements: Regular calibration of audiometers ensures that hearing measurements are accurate and consistent. Properly calibrated audiometers provide reliable results, which is essential for early detection of hearing problems and making appropriate clinical decisions.

Compliance with standards and regulations: Audiometers must comply with specific standards and regulations set by health agencies and regulatory bodies. Regular calibration is a requirement to meet these standards and ensure that the equipment conforms to established performance criteria.

Comparability of results: Calibration of audiometers ensures that results obtained at different times and locations are comparable with each other. This is especially important in longitudinal studies or in work environments where periodic hearing evaluations are performed to monitor the hearing health of workers.

Patient confidence: Proper calibration of audiometers provides confidence to both healthcare professionals and patients. Patients are confident that audiometric tests performed with properly calibrated equipment reflect their true hearing ability, which contributes to better medical care and informed decision making.

Maintaining equipment integrity: Regular calibration not only ensures measurement accuracy, but also helps to identify potential problems or deviations in audiometer performance. This allows timely corrective action to be taken and the proper integrity and functionality of the equipment to be maintained. audiometer calibration is essential to ensure accurate and reliable hearing measurements. It contributes to early detection of hearing problems, regulatory compliance, comparability of results, patient confidence and proper equipment maintenance. It is recommended to follow the manufacturer's guidelines and calibration standards established by recognized bodies to maintain the quality and accuracy of audiometers.

High frequency audiometry

High-frequency audiometry is a test used to evaluate a person's hearing ability in higher frequency ranges than what is evaluated in conventional audiometry.

While conventional audiometry generally evaluates frequencies between 250 Hz and 8,000 Hz, high-frequency audiometry can evaluate frequencies up to 20,000 Hz.This test is useful for detecting hearing loss in high frequencies, which may be especially important for the perception of high-pitched sounds and consonants in speech. Exposure to loud noises, age and some medical conditions can affect hearing in these higher frequencies.During high-frequency audiometry, special headphones or loudspeakers that emit high-frequency tones are used. The patient must indicate when he/she hears each tone, either with a button or by raising the hand. The results are recorded in an audiogram, which shows the patient's hearing at different frequencies.It is important to note that high frequency audiometry is not routinely performed in all hearing examinations, but is used in specific cases when high frequency hearing loss is suspected or when a more detailed assessment of hearing ability in these frequency ranges is desired.It is recommended to perform in cases of users exposed to noise, a chemical hazards and a history of repeated otitis media .

NRR hearing protectors

Hearing protectors are devices designed to protect the ears of workers and others from exposure to high noise levels. These devices reduce the amount of sound reaching the ear, helping to prevent noise-induced hearing loss and other related hearing problems. Here are some common types of hearing protectors:Ear plugs: These are small devices that are inserted into the ear canal. They can be made of foam, silica, wax or moldable material. Earplugs provide a physical barrier that reduces the intensity of the sound entering the ear. They are portable, inexpensive and easy to use.Earmuffs: Also known as co pa type hearing protectors, these are devices that completely cover the ears and create a seal around them. They consist of a rigid shell and cushioned ear pads that provide a comfortable fit and effective noise reduction. The earmuffs are suitable for working environments with higher noise levels.Electronic hearing protectors: These hearing protectors use electronic technology to reduce noise and amplify safe sounds. They enable communication and sound perception while attenuating harmful noise. Some models also have features such as noise cancellation and Bluetooth connectivity.Custom hearing protectors: These hearing protectors are custom-made to fit the unique shape of each individual's ear. An impression is taken of the ear canal and a customized hearing protector is created. These offer a precise and comfortable fit, resulting in greater effectiveness in noise reduction.
When selecting hearing protectors, it is important to consider the level of noise to which you are exposed, the duration of exposure, comfort, necessary communication and the specific requirements of the work environment. It is also essential to follow the manufacturer's instructions for proper use and to keep hearing protectors clean and in good condition. In addition, it is essential to train workers on the importance of wearing hearing protectors and to promote a culture of hearing safety in the workplace.NRR (Noise Reduction Rating) is a numerical value used to indicate the noise reduction capability of a hearing protector. It specifies the number of decibels (d B) that the hearing protector is expected to reduce from the ambient noise level before it reaches the wearer's ear.
The NRR is based on laboratory tests conducted in accordance with standards established by the U.S. Environmental Protection Agency (EPA) and is expressed in decibels (dB). The higher the NRR number, the greater the noise reduction capability of the hearing protector. However, it is important to note that the NRR does not represent a realistic noise reduction in all working environments. In practice, noise reduction can be affected by several factors, such as the proper fit of the hearing protector, the type and frequency of the noise, the duration of exposure and the

individual characteristics of the user.In addition, it is essential to understand that NRR is a measure of noise reduction under ideal laboratory conditions and should not be interpreted as a guaranteed noise reduction in all situations. Therefore, it is important to follow the manufacturer's recommendations and receive professional guidance in selecting and using the appropriate hearing protectors based on the specific needs of the work environment and the type of noise to which you are exposed.In some countries, such as the United States, the NRR has been replaced by the Hearing Protection Rating System (HPD) based on the International Classification System (ICS). The SIC uses a numerical rating to indicate different levels of hearing protection based on the effective noise reduction expected at the user's ear. This rating takes into account factors such as the fit and efficiency of the hearing protector under actual conditions of use.

Tuning forks

Tuning forks are instruments used in hearing evaluation to measure hearing function and detect possible hearing problems. These instruments emit pure tones and are used in various audiometric tests. Here are some ways tuning forks are used in relation to hearing:Weber test: In the Weber test, a vibrating tuning fork is placed on the midline of the individual's head. The vibration of the tuning fork is transmitted through the skull bones and it is evaluated if sound is perceived equally or unevenly in both ears. This test can help determine whether there is a conductive hearing loss or a sensorineural hearing loss.Rinne's test: In Rinne's test, a tuning fork is used to compare air and bone sound perception. The tuning fork is placed on the mastoid (bone behind the ear) and then moved close to the external auditory canal. It tests whether the individual can hear the tuning fork sound more clearly through air or bone. This test helps differentiate between a conductive hearing loss and a sensorineural hearing loss. Diagnostic tuning forks: There are also special diagnostic tuning forks that emit tones with specificfrequencies. These tuning forks are used to evaluate hearing in tests such as bone conduction audiometry. They are placed at specific points, such as the mastoid or forehead, and the individual's ability to perceive the emitted tone is measured.Auditory training: Tuning forks can also be used in auditory training programs. They can be used to develop auditory skills, such as pitch discrimination or perception of sound direction. Tuning forks can help train and fine-tune the auditory system to improve sound perception and understanding.It is important to note that the use of tuning forks in hearing evaluation is usually complemented by other tests, such as tonal audiometry, to obtain a complete and accurate assessment of hearing. Hearing health professionals, such as audiologists and speech-language pathologists, are responsible for performing these tests and analyzing the results to determine a person's hearing health.

DISORDERS ASSOCIATED WITH HEARING LOSS IN THE WORKER

Hearing loss may be associated with various disorders and conditions. These disorders may be direct or indirect causes of hearing loss, or may coexist with hearing loss. Some common disorders associated with hearing loss include:Tinnitus: Tinnitus is characterized by the perception of sounds in the ear or head that have no external source. It may manifest as a ringing, buzzing, whistling, hissing or other sounds. Tinnitus can be caused by exposure to loud noises, injury to the ear, or ear diseases such as hearing loss.Vertigo and dizziness: Vertigo refers to a sensation of spinning or whirling motion, while dizziness may be associated with a feeling of imbalance or instability. Some forms of vertigo and dizziness, such as Ménière's disease, may be related to hearing loss.Genetic disorders: Some genetic disorders can cause hearing loss. For example, presbycusis, which is age-related hearing loss, may have a genetic predisposition. Other genetic disorders, such as Usher syndrome, Waardenburg syndrome and neurofibromatosis type 2, may also be associated with hearing loss.Autoimmune diseases: Some autoimmune diseases, such as Ménière's disease, otosclerosis and autoimmune inner ear disease, can cause hearing loss. These diseases are characterized by an abnormal immune response that affects the ear tissues and may result in hearing loss.Neurological disorders: Certain neurological disorders, such as multiple sclerosis and brain tumors, can affect hearing and cause hearing loss. These disorders may damage the structures of the central auditory system or the nerves that transmit auditory information to the brain.It is important to note that not all people with hearing loss will experience these associated disorders, and the relationship may vary from person to person.

-Diabetes and hypoacusis

The relationship between diabetes and hypoacusis, or hearing loss, has been the subject of research and an association between the two conditions has been observed. While not all people with diabetes experience hearing loss, studies have shown that people with diabetes have an increased risk of developing hearing problems compared to those without diabetes.

Diabetes can affect hearing in several ways:

Damage to blood vessels : Diabetes can damage the small blood vessels in the inner ear, which are responsible for supplying blood and oxygen to the hearing cells. Deterioration of these blood vessels can lead to decreased hearing function.

Nerve damage: Diabetes can also affect the peripheral nerves, including the auditory nerves. This can lead to diabetic neuropathy, which can manifest as hearing loss or hearing impairment.Increased susceptibility to noise injury: Some studies suggest that people with diabetes may be more susceptible to damage caused by exposure to excessive noise. This may be due to the negative effects diabetes has on blood vessels and nerves in the ear.It is important to note that diabetes-associated hearing loss generally affects both ears and tends to be gradual, worsening over time. In addition, diabetes-related hearing loss may be more pronounced at higher frequencies.Users with diabetes should have their complete audiological studies to rule out hearing problems. It is recommended that you consult a hearing health professional, such as a speech-language pathologist, to perform a complete hearing evaluation and determine if there is a hearing loss related to diabetes.In some cases, treatment of diabetes and control of blood sugar levels may help prevent or delay the progression of hearing loss. In addition, the use of hearing aids or other assistive listening devices may be recommended to improve hearing in case of hearing loss.

- **Hypertension and hypoacusis**

Arterial hypertension, or high blood pressure, has also been associated with hearing loss. While not all people with hypertension experience hearing problems, several studies have found a link between the two conditions.

Hypertension can affect hearing in different ways:

Damage to blood vessels: Hypertension can damage blood vessels throughout the body, including blood vessels in the inner ear.
The blood and oxygen supply to hearing cells can be compromised, which can lead to hearing loss.Risk of vascular disease: Hypertension is a risk factor for the development of vascular disease, such as atherosclerosis. Atherosclerosis is characterized by narrowing and hardening of the arteries, which can affect blood flow to the inner ear and lead to hearing loss.Stroke risk: Hypertension is also associated with an increased risk of stroke. Strokes can damage areas of the brain that are involved in hearing, which can result in hearing loss.It is important to note that the relationship between hypertension and hearing loss is not completely understood and may vary from person to person. In addition, other risk factors, such as age, genetics, exposure to loud noise and smoking, may also influence hearing loss.If you have hypertension and are experiencing hearing problems,it is recommended that you consult a hearing health professional, as a speech therapist who will guide you if you require the use of a hearing aids .

-Obesity and hypoacusis

There is evidence to suggest an association between obesity and hearing loss. Several studies have shown that people with obesity have a higher risk of developing hearing problems compared to those with a healthy weight.

Obesity can affect hearing in several ways:

Circulatory problems: Obesity is associated with poor blood circulation due to increased adipose tissue, which can affect the blood and oxygen supply to the inner ear. Lack of adequate blood supply can contribute to degeneration of hearing cells and lead to hearing loss.Chronic inflammation: Obesity is also associated with a chronic inflammatory state in the body. Chronic inflammation can adversely affect the health of tissues, including those of the inner ear, and contribute to the development of hearing loss.Metabolic factors: Some studies suggest that metabolic factors associated with obesity, such as insulin resistance and elevated blood lipid levels, may influence hearing function and contribute to hearing loss.It is important to note that the relationship between obesity and hearing loss is not linear and may be influenced by other factors such as age, genetics, exposure to loud noise and smoking.In addition, it is recommended to adopt a healthy lifestyle that includes a balanced diet, regular exercise and weight control to help minimize the risk of hearing loss associated with obesity. The use of hearing aids or other assistive listening devices may also be recommended in case of hearing loss.

The occupational noise map

A noise map is a graphical representation that shows the noise levels in different areas or points of a specific environment. The main purpose of a noise map is to visualize the distribution of noise in a given area and to identify the areas where noise levels are highest.A noise map is a useful tool for identifying the areas of greatest noise exposure and developing appropriate control and mitigation strategies. In addition, it can be used for compliance with noise-related regulations and standards in occupational and urban environments.The process of preparing a noise map generally involvesthe following stages:Data collection: Noise level measurements are made at different locations within the area of interest. These measurements can be carried out using specialized noise measurement equipment, such as sound level meters. Data analysis: The data collected is analyzed to determine noise levels at each location. This may involve calculating average, maximum and minimum noise values, as well as identifying the time periods when the highest noise levels occur.

Graphical representation: Using mapping software or visualization tools, noise levels are plotted on a graphical map. Noise levels are usually indicated by colors or contours, where more intense colors or closer contours indicate higher noise levels.Interpretation and analysis: The noise map is analyzed to identify areas where noise levels are highest and areas where noise levels are lowest. This can help identify noise sources, assess the impact of noise on the environment, and make informed decisions about necessary control and mitigation measures.Control and mitigation actions: Based on the information provided by the noise map, measures can be implemented to control and reduce noise levels in identified problem areas. These measures may include modifying equipment or processes, installing noise barriers, implementing noise control programs, and raising awareness of the importance of noise reduction.Acoustic trauma refers to hearing injury or damage that occurs due to exposure to loud or intense sounds. This type of hearing injury can occur suddenly, as in the case of an explosion or a sudden, extremely loud sound, or gradually, as a result of continued exposure to excessive noise levels.When acoustic trauma occurs, the sensory cells of the inner ear, known as hair cells, may be damaged or destroyed. These cells are responsible for converting sound vibrations into electrical signals that are transmitted to the brain for interpretation. Damage to these cells can result in temporary or permanent hearing loss, depending on the severity of the trauma and the duration of exposure to the damaging sound.

The symptoms of acoustic trauma may vary, but generally include:
• Temporary or permanent hearing loss in one or both ears.
• Ringing in the ears (tinnitus), which may be constant or intermittent.
• Sensation of fullness or pressure in the ears.
• Excessive sensitivity to sound (hyperacusis), where the sounds are
may seem too strong or uncomfortable.

It is important to take measures to prevent acoustic trauma, especially in noisy environments or in situations where there is a risk of exposure to loud sounds. Some preventive measures include:Use hearing protection, such as earplugs or ear protectors, in noisy environments or during noisy activities, such as concerts, sporting events or the use of noisy tools and machinery.Keep the volume of music or audio devices at a safe level and avoid listening to music at high volumes through headphones or earphones.Take regular breaks from exposure to loud noises and limit exposure time to intense sounds.Educate yourself about safe noise levels and associated risks. with prolonged exposure to loud sounds.

Risk maps in schools

School risk maps are tools that allow the identification and visualization of potential hazards and risks present in the school environment. These maps are a graphic representation of the different risk factors, such as unsafe infrastructures, heavy traffic areas, electrical hazards, areas prone to flooding, among others.The main objective of risk mapping in schools is to prevent accidents and promote a safe environment for students, teachers and administrative staff. By identifying and mapping risks, preventive and mitigation measures can be taken to minimize hazards and ensure the safety of the educational community.Some common steps in the elaboration of risk mapping in the schools are:Hazard identification: A thorough analysis of the school environment is conducted to identify potential hazards and risks present. This may include inspections of facilities, evaluation of electrical and water systems, review of emergency procedures, among others.Information gathering: Relevant information is gathered on the risks identified, such as technical data, records of previous accidents, inspection reports, among others.Hazard mapping: The location of the various hazards is graphically represented on a school plan or map. This may include the use of symbols or colors to identify the different types of hazards.Analysis and evaluation: An analysis is made of the risks identified, evaluating their probability of occurrence and their potential impact on people's safety. This makes it possible to prioritize the and focus efforts on those posing the greatest risks.Planning prevention and mitigation measures: Based on the risk analysis, specific measures are designed and planned to prevent and mitigate the identified hazards. This may include actions such as infrastructure repairs, implementation of safety signage, training in emergency procedures, among others.It is important to emphasize that risk mapping in schools should be a participatory process that involves the educational community, including principals, teachers, students and administrative personnel. The participation of all stakeholders provides a more complete picture of the risks and fosters commitment and shared responsibility for school safety. Risk maps in schools are a valuable tool for promoting safe educational environments and preventing accidents. Their regular updating and their integration into risk management plans contribute to maintaining an environment conducive to learning and the well-being of all members of the educational community.

Promoting a culture of prevention from schools

Educating children about risk prevention is fundamental to promoting their safety and well-being. Teaching children about potential hazards and how to prevent them gives them the tools they need to make safe decisions and avoid risky situations.Development of self-protection skills: Teaching children to identify and prevent risks allows them to develop self-protection skills. They learn to recognize dangerous situations, make safe decisions and act appropriately to avoid accidents or injuries. These skills will accompany them throughoutand help them cope safely with the risks they face in their lives. they can find.Forming safe habits: Instilling safety habits from an early age helps children internalize them and incorporate them into their daily lives. When risk prevention becomes a regular practice, it reduces the likelihood of children being exposed to dangerous situations or engaging in reckless behavior.Promoting personal responsibility: By teaching children to prevent risks, the message is being conveyed that they are responsible for their own safety. This fosters the development of self-management skills and autonomy, as they learn to assess risks, make appropriate decisions and take responsibility for their actions.Accident and injury prevention: Accidents and injuries are one of the leading causes of morbidity and mortality in childhood. Risk prevention from an early age helps to reduce the incidence of accidents and injuries, protecting the physical integrity and health of children.Formation of safety attitudes and values: Risk prevention from the earliest years of life contributes to the formation of attitudes and values related to safety. Children learn to value and prioritize their own well-being as well as that of others. They internalize the importance of taking care of themselves and taking precautionary measures to avoid dangerous situations.Risk prevention from an early age is essential to protect the safety and well-being of children. It provides them with the necessary tools to safely face the challenges they may encounter throughout their lives, promoting responsible attitudes and safe habits. In addition, risk prevention from early childhood contributes to the reduction of accidents and injuries, safeguarding children's health and quality of life.Here are some strategies for educating children in prevention of risks:

1. Identify common hazards: Teach them to recognize the most common hazards in their environment, such as traffic, sharp objects, toxic products or water hazards. Help them understand the consequences of these hazards and how they can avoid them.
2. Encourage open communication: Establish a trusting environment where children feel safe to talk about the risks they face. Encourage children to ask questions and express their concerns. This will enable them to get appropriate information and guidance on how to avoid dangerous situations.

3. Educating children about risk prevention is fundamental to promoting their safety and well-being. Teaching children about potential hazards and how to prevent them gives them the tools they need to make safe decisions and avoid risky situations. Here are some strategies for educating children about risk prevention:

4. Identify common hazards: Teach them to recognize the most common hazards in their environment, such as traffic, sharp objects, toxic products or water hazards. Help them understand the consequences of these hazards and how they can avoid them.

5. Encourage open communication: Establish a trusting environment where children feel safe to talk about the risks they face. Encourage children to ask questions and express their concerns. This will enable them to get appropriate information and guidance on how to avoid dangerous situations.

6. Teach basic safety measures: Teach children basic safety measures, such as crossing the street safely, wearing seat belts in vehicles, not talking to strangers, and avoiding contact with hot or sharp objects. Explain the importance of following these guidelines to protect their safety.

7. Role-play: Role-play where children can practice how to act in risky situations. For example, can simulate a fire situation and practice how to safely exit a building. These activities will help them develop practical skills and make quick decisions in case of an emergency.

8. Use of educational resources: Use age-appropriate educational resources, such as picture books, videos and interactive games, that address risk prevention topics. These resources can help children better understand safety concepts and measures.

9. Visits to places of interest: Organize visits to places of interest related to safety, such as fire stations or health centers, where children can learn about the importance of risk prevention and obtain information from professionals in the field.

10. Personal example: Be a good role model by practicing safety measures in your own life. Children tend to imitate adult behavior, so if they see you taking precautions and following safety rules, they are more likely to do so as well.

Remember to adapt strategies and teachings to the children's age and level of understanding. Risk prevention education is a continuous and gradual process that should be reinforced on an ongoing basis so that children acquire solid risk prevention skills and knowledge.

Cellular damage by noise

Continuous or repeated exposure to high noise levels can have detrimental effects on the auditory cells of the inner ear, which can result in cell damage and hearing loss. This type of damage is known as acoustic trauma and can occur in the work environment as well as in recreational situations or exposure to intense noise. Prolonged loud noise can cause the release of harmful chemicals in the inner ear, which in turn can affect the sensory cells in the ear known as hair cells. These cells are responsible for converting sound waves into electrical signals that the brain can interpret as sound. When damaged, they can cause permanent hearing loss. Cell damage due to noise can manifest itself in different ways: Noise-induced hearing loss (NIHL): A common form of hearing loss caused by prolonged exposure to loud noise. It usually affects the high frequencies first and then spreads to lower frequencies. Tinnitus: Loud noise can trigger the appearance of ringing, buzzing or other sounds in the ears, known as tinnitus. This can be temporary or chronic and can be a symptom of cell damage in the inner ear. It is important to note that sensitivity to noise and susceptibility to damage can vary from person to person. Some people may experience cell damage and hearing loss even at lower exposure levels, while others may be more resistant. To prevent cell damage from noise, it is essential to follow hearing safety practices, such as wearing appropriate hearing protection in noisy environments, staying away from sources of excessive noise, limiting exposure to intense noise, and performing periodic hearing evaluations to detect any changes or deterioration. In addition, occupational regulations and standards often establish safe noise exposure limits in the work environment to protect workers' hearing health.

HEARING CONSERVATION PROGRAMS

The Occupational Safety and Health Administration (OSHA) in the United States establishes guidelines and regulations for hearing protection in the workplace. These guidelines include the implementation of hearing conservation programs to prevent and control noise-induced hearing loss in workers. The following are the key elements of hearing conservation programs according to OSHA:Noise Assessments: Employers must conduct noise assessments in the workplace to determine the exposure levels of workers. This involves measuring noise levels in different work areas and tasks using appropriate measuring instruments. Engineering controls: Engineering controls should be implemented to reduce noise levels at the source or in the transmission path. This may include the use of quieter machinery and equipment, noise barriers, noise insulation, and noise reduction techniques in facility design.Hearing protection program: Employers must establish a hearing protection program for workers exposed to hazardous noise levels. This involves providing adequate hearing protection, such as earplugs or earmuffs, and ensuring their correct and regular use.Training: Employers should provide training to workers on noise hazards, proper use of hearing protectors, safety procedures, and engineering controls in place. Training should also include information on the effects of noise on hearing and how to prevent hearing loss.Hearing surveillance program: Employers should offer hearing surveillance programs to monitor the hearing health of workers exposed to hazardous noise levels. This involves periodic audiometry to assess changes in hearing and take appropriate action if hearing loss is detected. Record keeping and documentation: Employers should maintain records and documentation of all noise assessments, engineering controls implemented, training provided, audiometric results, and any other relevant information related to hearing conservation.These are just some of the key elements that OSHA recommends for hearing conservation programs. However, it is important to note that specific regulations and guidelines may vary by country and jurisdiction. It is critical to comply with local regulations and to seek advice from occupational health and safety experts to ensure proper compliance with regulations and protect the hearing health of workers

Environmental health

Environmental health is a field of study that focuses on the effects of the environment on human health. Within this field, sound is an important environmental factor that can have a significant impact on human health. The following are some considerations on the relationship between environmental health and sound: Noise pollution: Excessive or unwanted sound, known as noise pollution or ambient noise, can have adverse effects on health. Prolonged exposure to high noise levels can cause stress, sleep disturbances, concentration problems, irritability and negatively affect psychological well-being. Effects on hearing: Intense and prolonged sound can damage the ears and cause hearing loss. Exposure to loud noise, such as constant vehicular traffic or industrial machinery, without adequate protection can be detrimental to hearing health. Impact on quality of life: Constant and disruptive noise can affect people's quality of life. It can interfere with daily activities, such as work, study, communication and rest, and generate generalized discomfort.Mental health effects: Chronic noise exposure has also been associated with mental health problems such as increased stress, anxiety, depression and mood disorders. In addition, it can affect concentration, cognitive performance and the ability to relax.Regulations and control measures: To protect people's health, regulations and standards related to noise pollution have been established in many countries. These regulations include noise exposure limits in different environments, such as residential areas, work spaces and public areas.It is important to take measures to reduce exposure to excessive noise and protect hearing health and general well-being. This may include the use of hearing protection in noisy environments, proper planning of urban areas to reduce noise exposure, and promoting awareness and education about the health effects of noise.

Vocology, the science of the voice

Vocology is a discipline concerned with the study and care of the human voice. While its primary focus is on the voice and voice-related disorders, it can also address issues related to noise and its impact on vocal health. The following are some considerations on the relationship between vocology and noise:Noise and vocal health: Excessive or prolonged noise can affect people's vocal health. Exposure to high levels of noise can cause vocal muscle strain, vocal cord irritation and overexertion when speaking or singing. This can lead to vocal problems such as dysphonia (voice disturbances), vocal fatigue, loss of vocal quality and increased risk of vocal injury.Voice use in noisy environments: People who work in noisy environments, such as teachers, singers in noisy places, or professionals who must speak in noisy environments, are at increased risk for vocal problems. The need to raise the voice to be heard in noisy environments can place increased stress on the vocal cords and increase the risk of vocal injuries or disorders. Preventive measures: To protect vocal health in noisy environments, a variety of preventive measures can be taken. These may include wearing hearing protection to reduce noise exposure, modifying environmental conditions to reduce background noise, implementing appropriate vocal amplification techniques to ensure healthy vocal projection, and learning vocal management techniques to help minimize vocal strain in noisy environments.Treatment of noise-related vocal disorders: In cases where noise has caused vocal problems, vocology professionals can provide vocal treatment and therapy to address the disorders and restore vocal health. This may include vocal rehabilitation techniques, training in healthy vocal production techniques, and guidelines for voice care and rest.Noise can have a negative impact on vocal health, and vocology plays an important role in the care and prevention of noise-related vocal disorders. By taking appropriate measures to reduce noise exposure and adopting healthy vocal practices, good vocal health can be maintained even in noisy environments.

High blood pressure and noise

Chronic exposure to noise, especially at elevated levels, has been associated with an increased risk of developing arterial hypertension. Some considerations on the relationship between noise and arterial hypertension are presented below: Stress and physiological response: Excessive and constant noise can generate a stress response in the body. Chronic stress can trigger a number of physiological responses, including the release of stress hormones such as cortisol and adrenaline, which can have adverse effects on the cardiovascular system.Sleep disturbance: Disturbing noise during the night can disrupt sleep and lead to insomnia problems. Sleep deprivation and reduced sleep quality have been associated with an increased risk of high blood pressure.Activation of the sympathetic nervous system: Exposure to intense noise can stimulate the sympathetic nervous system, which is responsible for the "fight or flight" response. This response can lead to an increase in heart rate, blood pressure and blood vessel contraction, which can contribute to the development of high blood pressure.Influence on health behaviors: Noise exposure can influence health behaviors such as physical activity, diet quality, and tobacco and alcohol consumption. These lifestyle factors are related to the development of high blood pressure.Long-term effects: Chronic exposure to noise over years can have a cumulative impact on cardiovascular health. Epidemiological studies have shown an association between the long-term exposure to traffic noise and increased risk of high blood pressure. It is important to note that the relationship between noise and arterial hypertension is complex and influenced by multiple factors. In addition, other risk factors for high blood pressure, such as age, gender, genetics, obesity, and family history, should also be considered in the risk assessment. However, it is recommended to take measures to reduce exposure to excessive noise and adopt an overall healthy lifestyle to prevent and control high blood pressure.

Noise and growth and development

Chronic noise exposure can have negative effects on the growth and development of individuals, especially children. The following are some considerations on the relationship between noise and growth:Interrupted sleep: Excessive noise during the night can disrupt sleep, which can negatively affect children's growth and development. Adequate sleep is essential for the production of growth hormones and for the repair and regeneration of body tissues.Chronic stress: Continued exposure to noise can lead to chronic stress in children. Chronic stress can have negative effects on growth and development, as it can affect the production of growth-related hormones and cause hormonal imbalances.Delayed cognitive development: Constant noise can affect children's ability to concentrate, academic performance and cognitive development. Chronic noise exposure in school environments can interfere with children's ability to process information and learn efficiently.Communication and language problems: Exposure to excessive noise can hinder communication and language development in children. Constant background noise can interfere with language acquisition, hindering children's ability to hear, process and produce language properly.Effects on the nervous system: Chronic exposure to noise can have negative effects on the developing nervous system of children. It can cause alterations in the auditory system and affect neuronal function, which can have implications for proper growth and development.It is important to take steps to reduce children's exposure to excessive noise, especially during critical periods of growth and development. This may include proper planning of school and home environments to reduce background noise, use of hearing protection in noisy situations, and promotion of healthy sleep practices. In addition, creating quiet, noise-free environments can promote optimal growth and development in children.

Noise and mental health

Chronic exposure to noise can have a significant impact on people's mental and emotional health, causing psychological harm. The following are some considerations on the relationship between noise and psychological harm:Chronic stress: Constant and disturbing noise can generate chronic stress in people. Chronic stress can trigger a physiological "fight or flight" response, increasing levels of stress hormones such as cortisol and adrenaline. This can negatively affect emotional and mental well-being and contribute to the development of anxiety disorders and depression.Difficulties with concentration and cognitive performance: Constant noise can interfere with concentration and cognitive performance. It can make it difficult to pay attention, process information information and memory, which can lead to frustration, irritability and decreased academic or work performance.Sleep disorders: Exposure to noise during the night can disrupt sleep and cause sleep disorders, such as insomnia. Insufficient or poor quality sleep can have a negative impact on mood, cognition and ability to cope with stress.Irritability and emotional distress: Chronic exposure to noise can lead to irritability, frustration and emotional distress. Constant noise can make it difficult to rest, relax and enjoy daily activities, which can affect mood and overall quality of life.Impact on mental health: Chronic noise exposure has been associated with an increased risk of developing mental disorders, such as anxiety disorders, mood disorders (such as depression) and sleep disorders. Constant noise can trigger and exacerbate these disorders in vulnerable individuals.It is important to take steps to reduce exposure to excessive noise and protect mental health. This may include the use of hearing protection, proper planning of environments to reduce noise, promoting healthy sleep practices, and adopting coping and relaxation strategies to counteract the effects of noise on psychological health.

MITIGATION OF NOISE

There are several measures that can be taken to mitigate noise and reduce its negative impact. Below are some common strategies and measures: Sound insulation: Improving the sound insulation of structures and spaces can help reduce the entry of outside noise. This involves the use of appropriate building materials, such as soundproof glazing and soundproof walls, as well as the installation of acoustic sealants and insulation in doors and windows.Sound barriers: The installation of sound barriers can help block and attenuate noise from external sources, such as roads or industry. These barriers can be natural, such as dense trees and shrubs, or artificial, such as sound-absorbing walls or panels. Use of hearing protectors: For those who are exposed to high noise levels in occupational or recreational settings, the use of hearing protectors, such as earplugs or noise-canceling headphones, can be an effective measure to reduce noise exposure and protect hearing.Regulation and urban planning: Local authorities can implement regulations and policies that limit noise exposure, especially in residential and sensitive areas such as schools and hospitals. In addition, proper urban planning can prevent the construction of noisy infrastructure near residential areas.Education and awareness: Education and awareness of the negative health effects of noise can help promote behavioral changes and encourage greater consideration for others in terms of noise. This includes promoting the use of quiet equipment and machinery, as well as respecting established noise limits in communities and neighborhoods.Quiet hours: Establishing quiet hours in residential and commercial areas can be an effective measure to reduce noise exposure during sleeping and resting hours.Green spaces and buffer areas: Creating and preserving green spaces and buffer areas between noise sources and residential areas can help reduce noise propagation and create quieter environments.It is important to consider that noise mitigation measures may vary depending on the context and the specific situation. It is advisable to consult with experts in acoustics or engineering to evaluate the needs and options available in each particular case.

HEALTH EDUCATION IN CONSTRUCTION

It is essential that health education in construction be continuous and regularly updated to address new risks and challenges that may arise in the sector. It must also be accessible to all workers, using effective methods of communication and adapted to the needs and characteristics of each group of workers.Health education in construction is critical to promoting the safety and well-being of construction workers. Below are some key areas on which health education in construction can be focused: Workplace safety: Education should focus on promoting workplace safety, including the correct use of personal protective equipment (PPE) such as hard hats,gloves, safety goggles, hearing protection, among others. Workers should receive training on the specific risks associated with construction, as well as on best practices to prevent accidents and injuries.Prevention of occupational diseases: Education should address the prevention of construction-related occupational diseases, such as exposure to asbestos, toxic chemicals, dust and other environmental contaminants. Workers should be informed about the risks and how to minimize exposure through measures such as the use of appropriate protective equipment, implementation of hygienic practices, and regular monitoring of their health.Ergonomics and prevention of musculoskeletal injuries: Education should include awareness of the importance of ergonomics in the workplace to prevent musculoskeletal injuries. Workers should receive information on proper posture, safe lifting, active breaks, and injury prevention techniques.Mental health and wellness: Construction health education should also address workers' mental health and wellness. This includes promoting awareness of work-related stress, anxiety and depression, as well as making supportive resources available and encouraging healthy and supportive work environments.Promotion of healthy lifestyles: Health education in construction can include the promotion of healthy lifestyles among workers, such as the importance of a balanced diet, regular physical activity, stress management and control of alcohol and tobacco consumption.

Risk prevention culture

Risk prevention culture refers to the values, beliefs, attitudes and practices that promote safety and risk prevention.accidents and illnesses in the workplace. It is a proactive approach that seeks to create a safe and healthy work environment, where risk prevention is a priority for all members of the organization. Some key aspects of the risk prevention culture include:Committed leadership: A culture of risk prevention begins with leadership committed to the safety and health of employees. Leaders must set a positive example by demonstrating their commitment to safety, actively participating in safety programs, encouraging employee

participation, and allocating the necessary resources to implement prevention measures.Employee participation: The risk prevention culture involves all employees in the identification and control of risks. Active employee participation in safety-related decision making, hazard identification, incident reporting, and implementation of preventive measures is encouraged. Employees should be encouraged to report unsafe conditions and suggest improvements.Effective communication: Clear and effective communication is essential to promote a culture of risk prevention. This includes providing clear information on existing risks, safety procedures, preventive measures and expectations for safe behavior. Communication should also be two-way, allowing employees to express their concerns and providing feedback on safety performance. Training and education: A culture of risk prevention is based on adequate training and education of employees regarding occupational hazards and preventive measures. Employees must receive the necessary training to understand the hazards associated with their work, as well as the best practices to prevent accidents and illnesses. Training should be ongoing and tailored to the specific needs of each worker.Recognition and rewards: Recognizing and rewarding employees for their commitment and contribution to safety and risk prevention can strengthen the culture of prevention. Recognition programs can include incentives, awards or simply verbal recognition and appreciation for safe practices.Continuous improvement:
The risk prevention culture involves a continuous improvement approach, where we seek to identify areas for improvement, learn from incidents and share lessons learned. Regular review of safety procedures, risk assessment and implementation of more effective preventive measures are encouraged.Fostering a culture of risk prevention requires a long-term commitment and the involvement of all levels of the organization. When safety becomes an integral part of an organization's culture, it creates a safer and healthier work environment for all its members.

Preventive planning of risks

Preventive risk planning refers to the identification, evaluation and control of occupational risks before they occur. It is a systematic process aimed at preventing or minimizing occupational accidents and illnesses, as well as promoting a safe and healthy work environment. Some key steps in preventive risk planning are as follows:Hazard identification: This step involves identifying potential hazards present in the workplace. This can be done through observation, analysis of previous incidents, review of safety reports and data, and consultation with employees. It is It is important to consider the different types of risks, such as physical, chemical, biological, ergonomic and psychosocial risks.Risk assessment: Once the risks have been identified, their possible consequences and the probability of their occurrence must be assessed. This involves assessing the severity of the potential harm, the exposure of workers to the risk and the probability of occurrence. Risk assessment can be based on qualitative or quantitative methods, and may require the use of tools such as checklists, risk matrices or safety analysis techniques.Risk control: After assessing the risks, appropriate control measures should be implemented to minimize or eliminate the identified risks. This may include the implementation of technical controls, such as physical barriers or ventilation systems, the adoption of administrative controls, such as safe work procedures and training, and the provision of appropriate personal protective equipment (PPE). It is important to follow the hierarchy of controls principle, which states that risks should be eliminated first, followed by risk reduction through control measures.Communication and training: During preventive risk planning, it is essential to clearly communicate the risks identified, the control measures implemented and the responsibilities of the workers. In addition, adequate training should be provided so that workers understand the risks and know how to work safely. Training should be ongoing and tailored to the needs of each worker.Follow-up and review: Risk prevention planning is not a static process, but requires regular review and follow-up. Mechanisms should be established to monitor the effectiveness of implemented control measures, identify new risk situations and make adjustments accordingly. Incident analysis and worker feedback are also important to continuously improve risk prevention planning.Preventive risk planning is essential to protect the safety and health of workers. By anticipating risks and taking proactive measures, you can create a safer work environment and prevent accidents and occupational illnesses. Risk factors can be classified into different categories, depending on their nature and origin. Below are some common classifications of risk factors:Physical risk factors: These factors refer to physical conditions in the work environment that may pose a risk to the health and safety of workers. Examples of physical risk factors include noise, vibration, radiation, extreme temperature, inadequate lighting, hazardous chemicals and sharp objects. Chemical risk factors: These factors relate to exposure to harmful chemicals in the workplace. They may include toxic gases, vapors, dusts, fumes, corrosive or flammable chemicals, and other hazardous materials. Exposure to chemicals can have acute or chronic effects on workers' health.Biological risk factors: These factors are related to exposure to biological agents, such as bacteria, viruses, fungi, parasites and other microorganisms. Workers exposed to these agents may be at risk of contracting infectious diseases, such as hepatitis, tuberculosis, influenza, among others. The health, agriculture and food industries are areas where biohazards may be encountered.Ergonomic risk factors: These factors refer to working conditions that can affect the musculoskeletal health and well-being of workers. They include intense physical strain, repetitive movements, awkward postures, inadequate workspace design, lack of breaks and rest periods, and manual handling of heavy loads. Ergonomic hazards can contribute toto the development of musculoskeletal disorders, such as back injuries, tendonitis and carpal tunnel syndrome. Psychosocial risk factors: These factors relate to the psychological and social aspects of work that can affect the mental and emotional health of workers. They include job stress, excessive workload, lack of control over tasks, harassment at work, lack of social support, job insecurity, and lack of work-life balance. Psychosocial factors can have a significant impact on the emotional well-being and mental health of workers.It is important to recognize and evaluate all these risk factors in the workplace in order to implement appropriate preventive measures and ensure a safe and healthy work environment.

The adolescent as worker

The adolescent worker refers to those young people who are in the adolescent stage and are employed, either in part-time or full-time jobs. This situation may arise for a variety of reasons, such as economic necessity, the desire for financial independence or the search for work experience.However, employment during adolescence raises certain specific considerations and challenges. Some relevant points are presented below:Labor legislation: Countries often have laws that regulate the employment of adolescents, establishing restrictions on the hours of work, the type of work allowed and the minimum age for employment. These laws are intended to protect young workers and ensure their safety and well-being.Balance between work and education: It is important for working adolescents to be able to balance their employment with their academic responsibilities. Formal education plays a role The work must not interfere negatively with their development and future, so it must be ensured that the work does not interfere negatively with their school performance.Health and safety: Employers and authorities must ensure the safety and well-being of adolescent workers. This involves providing a safe work environment, training them in safety practices, and ensuring that applicable labor standards are met.Personal and professional development: Work can be an opportunity for adolescents to acquire skills and experiences that will be useful to them in the future. It can also give them the opportunity to develop autonomy, responsibility and money management skills. Supervision and support: Working adolescents can benefit from adequate supervision and support from adults, such as their parents, guardians or employers. This involves providing guidance, emotional support and ensuring that they are not exploited or abused in the workplace. It is important to emphasize that work during adolescence must be compatible with their physical, emotional and educational development. Adolescents must have access to safe and adequate employment opportunities, and measures must be taken to prevent their exploitation or detriment.

Ultimately, it is critical to find a balance between work and other important aspects of a teenager's life, such as education, recreational activities and time to socialize with friends and family.

The working adult

Risk prevention in the workplace is crucial to ensure the safety and well-being of workers, including adults working in the food industry. construction. The following are some important considerations regarding risk prevention in the adult construction worker:Risk identification and assessment: It is essential to carry out a thorough assessment of the risks present in the construction work environment. This involves identifying the specific hazards associated with the tasks and activities performed, such as falls from heights, exposure to chemicals, risk of entrapment, among others. The risk assessment allows the implementation of appropriate preventive measures.Training and education: Construction workers must receive adequate training and education in occupational risk prevention. This includes knowledge of safe work procedures, proper use of personal protective equipment, safety measures specific to the construction industry, and proper handling of materials and tools. Ongoing training is key to keeping risk prevention knowledge up to date.Use of personal protective equipment (PPE): Construction workers must adequately and consistently use the appropriate personal protective equipment for their work. This may include hard hats, gloves, safety glasses, ear protectors, safety shoes, among others. Proper use of PPE helps to mitigate risks and protect the worker from potential injuries.Safe work organization: It is important to establish proper planning and efficient organization of construction work to minimize risks. This includes coordinating activities, marking hazardous areas, implementing safety protocols and taking measures to prevent accidents and injuries.Supervision and follow-up: Regular supervision by those responsible for occupational safety is essential to ensure that risk prevention standards are met and that the necessary measures are taken to protect workers. In addition, it is should conduct periodic follow-ups and reviews of work processes and conditions to identify possible safety improvements.Promoting a safety culture: It is essential to promote a safety culture in the construction industry, where risk prevention is a priority shared by all team members. This involves fostering open communication about safety, encouraging workers to report risk situations, and recognizing and valuing good practices in risk prevention. Risk prevention in the adult construction worker requires a comprehensive approach and commitment from both employers and workers. The implementation of adequate prevention measures contributes to reducing the incidence of accidents and injuries, and to providing a safe and healthy work environment in the construction industry.

Occupational anamnesis

Occupational history, also known as work history or occupational history, is an important part of an individual's occupational health and medical evaluation. It consists of collecting detailed information about an individual's work history and occupational exposures. The main objective of the occupational history is to identify the occupational hazards to which a person has been exposed, as well as to assess any possible relationship between work factors and current or past health conditions. During the occupational history taking, a health professional or occupational health specialist may ask questions related to the following aspects:Employment history: Details are collected on the person's previous and current employment, including duration, type of work performed, specific duties, etc.and potential exposures in each job. This may include exposure to chemicals, noise, vibrations, radiation, biological agents, extreme temperatures, ergonomically unfavorable postures, among others. Specific exposures: Inquiries are made about specific exposures in the work environment, such as chemicals, fumes, dusts, gases, solvents, pesticides or other toxic substances.History of work-related injuries: Information is collected on any work-related injuries or illnesses that have occurred in the past, such as accidents, musculoskeletal injuries, or exposures to toxic agents.Use of personal protective equipment (PPE): Evaluate whether PPE, such as helmets, goggles, ear protectors, masks, gloves, among others, have been used and are being used properly, according to the nature of the work and the exposures involved.Working conditions: Consideration is given to aspects related to the working environment, such as noise level, lighting, temperature, ventilation and ergonomics.Occupational anamnesis can provide valuable information for the assessment of occupational hazards, the diagnosis of work-related diseases and the implementation of preventive measures. It is important that individuals are honest and provide accurate information during this process, as this contributes to proper assessment and management of occupational hazards and occupational health.

The sound level meter

The sound level meter is a measuring instrument used to measure the sound pressure level, i.e. the volume or intensity of sound in the environment. It is designed to provide an objective measure of the noise level and is used in a variety of applications, including occupational risk assessment, noise pollution control, environmental impact studies and quality control in industry. The use of the sound level meter involves the following general steps:Preparation: Before using a sound level meter, it is necessary to perform an initial calibration to ensure that the device is correctly adjusted and providing accurate measurements. This is accomplished by using an acoustic calibrator, which emits a known reference tone. Configuration: The sound level meter should be configured according to the specific needs of the measurement. This includes setting the frequency weighting (A, C or Z), which allows the sound level meter response to be adapted to different frequency ranges. A-weighting is commonly used in environmental noise measurements, as it matches the sensitivity of the human ear.Positioning: The sound level meter is placed in the desired location for the measurement. It is important to make sure that the sound level meter microphone is correctly positioned and is not obstructed by objects that may alter the measurement.Measurement: Once the sound level meter is configured and positioned, the sound level measurement is performed. The sound level meter shows the sound pressure level value in decibels (dB) on its display. Depending on the configuration of the sound level meter, it can also record additional data, such as the maximum value, the minimum value and the time-weighted average.Interpretation of results: Measurement results may be interpreted in accordance with limits established by applicable regulations or standards. In some cases, permissible exposure levels may be established to protect human health and safety. Interpretation of results may also require consideration of additional factors, such as the duration of noise exposure.It is important to follow the sound level meter manufacturer's instructions and to have the proper training to use the meter correctly. This ensures accurate and reliable measurements, which is essential for assessing and controlling noise-related hazards and hearing protection.

TYPE

There are several types of sound level meters available, designed for different applications and measurement needs. The following are some of the most common types of sound level meters:Integrating Sound Level Meters: These sound level meters measure and record sound pressure level as a function of time. They can provide average, maximum and minimum noise level measurements, and generally have the ability to store data for later analysis. They are widely used in environmental impact studies, industrial noise assessments and environmental noise measurements.Real-Time Sound Level Meters: These sound level meters display sound pressure level measurements in real time, allowing immediate visualization of the data. They are useful for real-time noise monitoring and field measurements. They can also include additional functions, such as frequency analysis and audio recording.Two Channel Sound Level Meters: Two channel sound level meters have the ability to simultaneously measure the sound level at two different locations or apply different frequency weightings to each channel. They are useful in applications where it is required to compare sound levels at different locations or when different frequency bands need to be measured separately.Octave and Frequency Band Sound Level Meters: These sound level meters have the ability to analyze and display measurements in specific frequency bands. Octave sound level meters measure in octaves and frequency band sound level meters measure in narrower bands, such as thirds of an octave. They are useful in applications where the frequency content of sound needs to be analyzed, such as in the evaluation of the acoustic quality of interior spaces or in the design of acoustic insulation systems. Dosimeter Sound Level Meters: Dosimeter sound level meters are used to measure personal noise exposure over a given period of time. These devices are commonly used in occupational risk assessments to measure an individual's cumulative noise dose over the course of a workday. They provide information on average exposure and cumulative exposure as a function of time.It is important to note that different types of sound level meters may have specific features and capabilities depending on the model and manufacturer. When selecting a sound level meter, it is advisable to evaluate the specific measurement needs and ensure that the device meets the standards and requirements applicable to the intended application.

OCCUPATIONAL HEALTH AUDITS

An occupational health audit is a systematic and objective process to evaluate and verify compliance with occupational health and safety standards, regulations and best practices in the workplace. The main objective of an occupational health audit is to identify deficiencies, risks and areas for improvement in an organization's occupational health and safety management system.The occupational health audit process may vary according to the specific needs and requirements of each organization, but generally involves the following steps:Audit planning: The scope and objectives of the audit are established, the audit team is determined, and the schedule and resources needed to conduct the audit are planned.Information gathering: Relevant information is gathered on the organization's occupational health management system, including policies, procedures, records, incident and risk reports, and any other relevant documentation.On-site assessment: A site visit is conducted to directly assess working conditions, personal protective equipment, risk identification and assessment, compliance with applicable standards and regulations, personnel training and other areas related to occupational health and safety.Interviews and consultations: Interviews are conducted with the organization's personnel, including employees, supervisors and managers, to obtain a more complete understanding of occupational health-related practices and procedures. Consultations may also be conducted with employee representatives and other relevant stakeholders.Analysis and evaluation of findings: Audit findings are analyzed and evaluated against established criteria, such as regulations, industry standards and best practices. Gaps, deficiencies and areas for improvement in the occupational health management system are identified.Audit report: A detailed report is prepared documenting the audit findings, observations and recommendations. The report may include a description of strengths and areas for improvement, as well as a recommended action plan to address identified deficiencies.Follow-up and corrective action: Once the audit report is issued, a follow-up is carried out to verify the implementation of the recommended corrective actions. Progress is monitored and improvements made to the occupational health management system are followed up. An occupational health audit can be performed by internal personnel of the organization or by external auditors, such as consultants specialized in occupational health. The audit provides organizations with an objective assessment of their OHS performance, enabling them to identify areas for improvement and strengthen their management system to ensure a safe and healthy working environment for employees.

WHAT IS REVIEWED IN A CLINICAL AUDIT IN OCCUPATIONAL HEALTH?

Clinical audits can be conducted by professionals internal to the healthcare organization or by external auditors, such as quality and patient safety experts. The results of clinical audits are used to identify opportunities for improvement, implement changes in care processes, and ensure quality and safe care for workers.Clinical audits are a systematic and objective process conducted to assess the quality of care and ensure compliance with standards, protocols and best clinical practices in a healthcare setting. The primary objective of clinical audits is to improve the quality of care and patient safety by identifying areas for improvement and ensuring compliance with established standards.Clinical audits can cover different aspects of occupational health care, such as:Clinical procedures and protocols: The clinical procedures and protocols used in the diagnosis, treatment and follow-up of patients are reviewed and evaluated. This includes verifying whether evidence-based best practices are being followed and whether there is compliance with established standards.Documentation: Health documentation, such as medical records, laboratory reports, radiology reports, among others, are analyzed to ensure that they are complete, accurate and comply with legal and regulatory requirements. It also verifies whether the information is being recorded in an adequate and timely manner. Worker safety: The implementation of worker safety measures, such as correct identification of the user, prevention of work-related infections, safe administration of medications by the physician, and prevention of falls or other adverse events are evaluated.Regulatory compliance: Compliance with the rules and regulations established by the relevant health agencies is verified. This may include regulations on privacy and confidentiality of patient data, licensing and accreditation requirements, and risk management policies. Outcomes and clinical performance: Treatment outcomes and clinical performance indicators are analyzed to assess the effectiveness of clinical procedures and care provided. This may include treatment success rate, waiting time for care, patient satisfaction and other relevant indicators. Education and training: The level of knowledge and competence of the medical and nursing staff is assessed through review of their credentials, certifications and continuing education records. Adequate education and training programs are being implemented to maintain and improve care skills.

INFORMED CONSENT FORM

1. Please read the following form with the information below carefully before deciding to participate in the research study.

I am currently a licensed speech pathologist; as a requirement, a case study will be carried out in order to learn about the sign-symptomatology of hearing impairment. The information obtained through this study will be kept under strict confidentiality and your name will not be used. There will be no any breach of confidentiality as required by law. You have the right to withdraw consent for participation at any time. There is no risk involved in the case study; as long as the speech-language pathologist handles the procedures correctly. You will receive no compensation for participation other than the courtesy of therapeutic care. You may contact me at my cell phone number is   and e-mail

2. This form describes in simple language what the subject of the study does.

The patient will be evaluated once the existence of a hearing deficit is confirmed, indicating the diagnosis. Within the evaluations, the patient will be asked to answer questions inherent to his/her lifestyle and personal conditions that may at any given time have an impact and/or the conditions for which he/she is referred. Subsequently, a series of procedures and strategies will be established in order to assess the hearing conditions, so as to contribute to the topodiagnosis of the pathology. It is reiterated that there will be no risk, however if there are clinical situations arising from negligence in audiological care, free care will be provided until the conditions are corrected. There will be no indemnities, not even for the patient who is filmed and photographed during the examination to be submitted for diagnosis.

After having read, understood and clarified all the information provided to the research protocol procedures, I decide to participate voluntarily as a case study subject.

Name of research subjectSignature of person in charge ID y Link

Name of researcherSignature of researcher ID

BIBLIOGRAPHY

Alfie Cohen, M., & Salinas Castillo, O. (2017). Noise in the city. Hearing pollution and walkable city. Demographic and urban studies, 32(1), 65-96.

Álvarez Heredia, F. (2007). Occupational health.

Álvarez, F., Conti, L., Valderrama, F., Moreno, O., & Jiménez, I. (2011). Salud occupational. Ecoe Ediciones.

Amén Chinga, S. G. (2016). Design and application of the auditory conservation program for the prevention of alterations of workers occupationally exposed to noise of the heavy equipment and turbine departments of the Empresa Pública de Hidrocarburos del Ecuador del Cantón Shushufindi provincia de Sucumbíos (Master's thesis, Riobamba: Universidad Nacional de Chimborazo, 2015).

Andrade Ruíz, C. O. (2009). Evaluation of the risk of occupational hearing loss and implementation of a hearing conservation program in the company Ekador SA (Bachelor's thesis, Quito: Universidad de las Américas, 2009).

Arosemena, A.R.(2014).Salud occupational, researchy pathologies Professional. Medicine, 18(3).

Badía Montalvo, R. (1985). Occupational health and occupational hazards. Bulletin of the Pan American Sanitary Bureau (PASB); 98 (1), Jan. 1985.

Bello, M. D. C. M. (1995). Effects of noise from occupational exposure. Health of the Workers, 3(2), 93-101.

Calzaretta, A. V., Valenzuela, L. V., & Sepúlveda, F. M. (2010). The study of risk perception and occupational health: a look from risk paradigms. Science & Work, 12(35).

Campos Ramiro (2022). Audiological dictionary, A practice from audiology, 22(3). Spanish academic publishing house

Dreossi, R. C. F., & Momensohn-Santos, T. (2005). O ruído e sua interferência sobre estudantes em uma sala de aula: revisão de literatura. Pró-Fono Revista de Atualização Científica, 17, 251-258.

De los Ángeles Aguilera-Velasco, M., Fernández, M. A., Figueroa, R. M. R., Figueroa, M. G. M., & Radillo, B. E. P. (2008). Socioeducational intervention and promotion of Occupational Health. Cuban Journal of Health and Work, 9(2), 50-60.

Farfán, C., Leviante, R., & Solís, F. (2005). HIGH-FREQUENCY HEARING IN SUBJECTS EXPOSED TO NOISE. Revista Chilena de Tecnología Médica, 25(1).

García Ortiz, M. J., Torres Núñez, M. M., Torres Fortuny, A., Alfonso Muñoz, E., & Cruz Sánchez, F. (2017). High-frequency audiometry: usefulness in the audiological diagnosis of noise-induced hearing loss. Revista Archivo Médico de Camagüey, 21(5), 584-591.

Hällgren, M., Larsby, B., & Arlinger, S. (2006). A Swedish version of the Hearing In Noise Test (HINT) for measurement of speech recognition: A Swedish version of the Hearing In Noise Test (HINT) for assessment of speech recognition. International Journal of Audiology, 45(4), 227-237.

Grass Martínez, Y., Castañeda Deroncelé, M., Pérez Sánchez, G., Rosell Valdenebro, L., & Roca Serra, L. (2017). Noise in the stomatological work environment. Medisan, 21(5), 527-533.

Hernández Díaz, A., & González Méndez, B. M. (2007). Auditory alterations in workers exposed to industrial noise. Medicina y Seguridad del Trabajo, 53(208), 09-19.

Hernández-Gaytán, S. I., Santos-Burgoa, C., Becker-Meyer, J. P., Macías-Carrillo, C., & López-Cervantes, M. (2000). Prevalence of hearing loss and correlated factors in a cement industry. public health of mexico, 42(2), 106- 111.

Kuna, H. D., García Martínez, R., & Villatoro, F. (2009). Information Exploitation Procedures for the Identification of Missing, Noisy and Inconsistent Data. In XI Workshop of Researchers in Computer Science.

Pino Díaz, F. E. (2016). Evaluation of occupational noise and development of a hearing conservation plan for workers at the Alao hydroelectric power plant in the province of Chimborazo (Bachelor's thesis, Quito: Universidad de las Américas, 2016).

Machado, C. S. S. S., Valle, H. L. B. D. D. S. D., Paula, K. M. D. D., & Lima, S. D. S. (2011).
Characterization of the auditory processing of children with reading and writing disorders from 8 to 12 years old under treatment at the Centro Clínico de Fonoaudiologia da Pontifícia Universidade Católica de Minas Gerais. Revista CEFAC, 13, 504-512.

Ramírez, A. V. (2012, January). Occupational health services. In Annals of the Faculty of Medicine (Vol. 73, No. 1, pp. 63-69). UNMSM. Faculty of Medicine.

Rivera La Rosa, J. R., & Gamarra Carpio, J. C. (2020). Threshold changes in audiometry according to Osha and Niosh criteria in noise-exposed workers of an industrial company from 2013 to 2018.

Ruiz Casal, E., Campos, M. E., López Campos, D., & Pérez Piñero, B. (2000). High-frequency audiometry: thresholds in relation to age. ORL-DIPS, 165- 167.

Sauvage, J. P., Puyraud, S., Roche, O., & Rahman, A. (2000). Anatomy of the ear in-house. EMC-Otorhinolaryngology, 29(1), 1-19.

Salcedo Pino, M. G., & Cuno Palomino, H. W. (2022). Evaluation of noise levels for the implementation of a hearing conservation program in the ore processing plant of the company Gold Processing & Research Group SAC.

Sguassero, J. (1999). Exploratory study on noise pollution and effects

Noise Harmful to Individuals, Rosario, 1998.

Thomassin, J. M., & Barry, P. (2016). Anatomy and physiology of the external ear. EMC- Otolaryngology, 45(3), 1-13.

Valiente, A. R., Fidalgo, A. R., Villarreal, I. M., & Berrocal, J. R. G. (2016). Audiometry with extension at high frequencies (9,000-20,000 Hz). Usefulness in audiological diagnosis. Acta Otorrinolaringológica Española, 67(1), 40-44.

Zamberlan-Amorim, N. E., Fujinaga, C. I., Hass, V. J., Fonseca, L. M. M., Fortuna, C. M., & Scochi, C. G. S. (2012). Impact of a participatory noise reduction program in a neonatal unit. Revista Latino-Americana de Enfermagem, 20, 109-116.

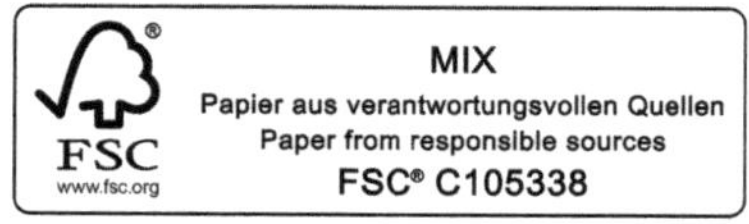

Printed by Books on Demand GmbH, Norderstedt / Germany